Z GRILLS

WOOD PELLET GRILL & SMOKER

COOKBOOK FOR BEGINNERS

HEALTHY & NATURAL RECIPES TO KEEP FIT AND MAINTAIN ENERGY

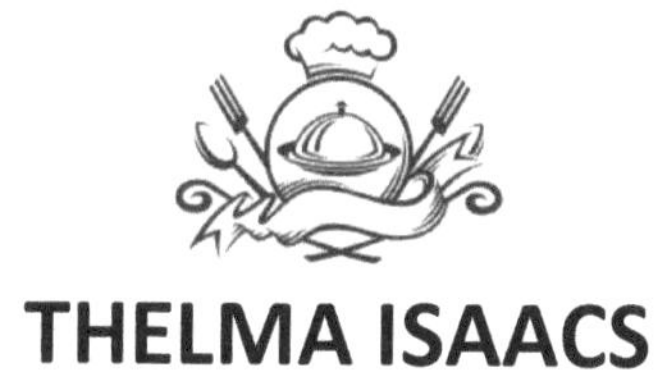

THELMA ISAACS

CONTENTS

INTRODUCTION

What the Z Grills Wood Pellet Grill is

A wood pellet grill — also known as a wood pellet smoker — is a special type of grill that uses indirect, pellet-generated heat and smoke to cook food in several different ways. With a pellet grill, you can enjoy traditionally grilled favorites or leave the meat to cook slowly on low smoke throughout the day. You can also use a pellet grill like a type of outdoor oven.

Like other grills, a pellet smoker makes an excellent addition to a campout, tailgating party and your own backyard.

How Does the Z Grills Wood Pellet Grill Work?

So now you know what they do, but how do pellet grills work?

Much of what a pellet grill does is automated, meaning there's a very small learning curve on figuring out how to operate it correctly. Wood pellets are loaded into a storage chamber called the hopper, where a motor and combustion fan ignite the pellets and circulate that smoky wood flavor throughout the main cooking chamber.

Once they're going, pellet grills work basically like a gas grill or kitchen oven, trapping heat under the hood to cook your food, all while the hopper continues to circulate the aroma and flavor of your choice of wood pellets. Air fans ensure that heat and smoke are evenly dispersed during the cook time, and temperature control dials give you the option to cook either low and slow or hard and fast, depending on the taste and texture that you're trying to achieve.

The Pros of the Z Grills Wood Pellet Grill

1.   Laid-Back Approach

If you're not the type of person to babysit your grill, opting for a pellet grill can be a far better option. Compared to gas, pellet grills cook slowly and thoroughly with minimal intervention and safety concerns. You'll even find that many have easy-to-use features that allow you to monitor the cooking process remotely.

For example, some pellet grills are equipped with digital controllers that allow you to set specific cook times. You can even use a smartphone app to adjust the grill settings. The only maintenance you'll have to consider with a wood pellet grill vs propane grill is making sure the hopper has enough pellets.

2. Minimal Maintenance

Because pellet grills typically cook for longer, most of the fats and grease will be burnt away, compared to gas grills. At most, you'll have to clean the firepot and any juices and drippings that are collected. You could also opt to season the smoker after cooking to burn away any traces of food.

3. Superior Flavor

The number one reason why people suggest pellet grills are better than gas grills is their flavor profiles. With pellet grills, you will have a diverse selection of different types of wood that you can cook with.
Instead of using regular flavorless gas, these appliances allow you to inject different flavors into the meat. A few of the most popular flavored pellets on the market include pecan, mesquite, hickory, and apple. There are plenty of manufacturers that have an extensive product list of fabulously flavored wood pellets. If you buy them in bulk, you're likely to get better discounts than you would with gas canisters.
Another exciting aspect of the flavors from wood pellets is you can customize them to your liking. You could mix apple and mesquite pellets for a unique flavor for ribs and brisket.

4. Versatility

Interestingly enough, pellet grills are far more versatile than gas grills because they give you several different ways to cook. You can easily set the temperature low, close the lid for smoking, or use it as a traditional grill. Some of the higher-end models even allow you to sear and braise, as well.

5. Enhanced Moisture and Meat Quality

Most people who opt for gas grills search for a quick and efficient outdoor appliance for everyday meals. With a pellet smoker, you have more control over how your meat cooks, especially if you want juicier cuts.
Since this appliance cooks for longer times and at lower temperatures, you'll find the inside of meat will be more moist. You might also find that it's a preferable option for higher-quality cuts of meat that need more attention.

Better to Use Your Z Grills Wood Pellet Grill

1. Use Lighter-Flavored Wood

Switching up your hardwood changes the flavor of what you're cooking.

You'll want to leave the big smoke flavors for meat and veggies and use a lighter-flavored wood for your baked goods.

You simply want the wood flavor to lightly touch your baked goods. Go ahead and experiment to see which flavors you like the best. Go ahead and combine them, too.

2. Prep Your Ingredients

Just like with baking in the house, you want to prep your ingredients ahead of time. Then, put it all together so it's ready to cook when you are.

For example, if you're having an evening party, put your dessert together in the morning, so you just have to slip it into your grill when you're ready to cook.

3. Keep It Simple

Whether you're a novice baker or a seasoned expert, let the flavor of your hardwood season your baked goods and give it a light smoky flavor.

So, keep your dessert simple and let the grill do the work. There's no reason to over complicate your dessert. After all, the fun of having a party is hanging out with friends and family.

Think cookies, cake, crumbles, and even fruit. Grilled fruit is delightful and refreshing when you put some cool whip on the side.

4. Use a Recipe You Know

A great tip is to use a recipe you know and are comfortable with. You can basically make anything you'd like on your pellet grill. So, pull out your favorite cookie, brownie, cake, pie, or cheesecake recipe. You don't really have to make any modification to cook on your grill.

Do note, though, that recipes may cook a bit faster, so you'll want to check often for doneness.

Cleaning Approaches for Your Z Grills Wood Pellet Grill

To prove to you just how easy it can be let's review the common methods of cleaning.

1. The Obvious Approach: Brushing

This method works best if it is done immediately after grilling while the grate is still hot. Before the grates cool off, scrape each grate with a brush, both top and bottom sides. You can also dip the brush in water which will create a steam that loosens the grease. Not only will this make cleaning time shorter, but it will discourage insects from hanging around your grill. Depending on your grate you may need to wipe them down with a cloth after scrapping.

2. The Lazy Approach: Burning

The idea behind this method is simple, get the grate super hot (550° F) until all the caked on grease burns up. You can throw the grates in a self-cleaning oven or simply place some aluminum foil down on top of the grate, close the lid and light up the grill. After about 10-15 minutes all of the grease should be a white powder, simply brush it off and you're done.

3. The Neat Freak Approach: Soaking

Although, brushing and burning are the standard methods for cleaning, all grates should be soaked at least a couple times a year.

Just fill up the sink or a large bucket with water and a bunch of dish soap. Add a little baking soda and let the grates soak for an hour. Afterward, scrub and rinse.

4. The DIY Approach

You can easily make your own scrubber with a block of hardwood. Use the block to scrub the grates after grilling, eventually, you will carve grooves into the block that fit perfectly onto your grate.

Aluminum foil is another easy DIY scrubber and also a lifesaver if you have to use a lazy person's grill. Simply heat up the grates, then wad up some foil and scrub away. Let's jump into some do-it-yourself methods to cleaning up those nasty grates.

BAKING RECIPES

Baked Cheesy Parmesan Grits

Servings: 4
Cooking Time: 60 Minutes

Ingredients:
- 4 Cup chicken stock
- 3 Tablespoon butter
- 3/4 Teaspoon salt
- 1 Cup quick grits
- 1 Cup shredded cheddar cheese
- pepper
- 1/2 Cup Monterey Jack cheese, shredded
- 1/2 Cup whole milk
- 2 Large eggs

Directions:

1. Supply your smoker with wood pellets and follow the start-up procedure. Preheat the grill, with the lid closed, to 350° F.

2. Butter an 8" baking dish or a 10" cast iron pan.

3. Bring the chicken stock, butter, and salt to boil in medium saucepan. Gradually whisk in grits.

4. Reduce heat to medium and cook until mixture thickens slightly, stirring often about 8 minutes. Remove from heat.

5. Add cheeses and stir until melted. Season with pepper and salt to taste.

6. Whisk together milk and eggs in small bowl. Gradually whisk mixture into grits.

7. Pour the cheese grits into the buttered cast iron pan. Bake until grits feel firm to touch, about 1 hour. Grill: 350 °F

8. Remove from grill and let stand 10 minutes before serving. Enjoy!

Crème Brûlée

Servings: 2
Cooking Time: 45minutes

Ingredients:
- 1 Quart heavy whipping cream
- 1 Pieces Vanilla Bean, split and scraped
- 6 Large egg yolk
- 1 Cup sugar

Directions:

1. Supply your smoker with wood pellets and follow the start-up procedure. Preheat the grill, with the lid closed, to 325° F.

2. Pour the cream into a saucepan over medium-high heat, add the vanilla bean and the scraped seeds. Bring to a boil. Remove from the heat and allow to steep (about 15 minutes). Remove the vanilla bean from saucepan and discard.

3. In a bowl, whisk together egg yolks and 1/2 cup (100 g) of the sugar until the mix starts to lighten in color. Add the cream a little at a time, stirring continually.

4. Pour the mixture into 6 (8 oz) ramekins and place the ramekins into a large roasting pan. Pour hot water into the pan so that it comes halfway up the sides of the ramekins.

5. Place water bath pan on the grill and bake until the Crème Brûlées still jiggle in the center, about 40 to 45 minutes. Grill: 325 °F

6. Remove the ramekins from the roasting pan and refrigerate for at least 2 hours and up to 2 days.

7. To serve, let the Crème Brûlée come to temperature (about 20 minutes) before torching the tops.

8. Sprinkle the remaining 1/2 cup (100 g) sugar equally on top of each ramekin. Using a torch in a circular motion, melt the sugar until it caramelizes and forms a crispy top.

9. Allow the Crème Brûlée to sit for a few minutes before serving. Enjoy!

Baked Potatoes & Celery Root Au Gratin

Servings: 2
Cooking Time: 60 Minutes

Ingredients:
- 5 Tablespoon butter, softened
- 2 Large leeks, white parts only, cleaned and sliced into half moons
- kosher salt
- freshly ground black pepper
- 5 Small Yukon Gold potatoes, sliced 1/4 inch thick
- 2 Whole celery root, peeled and sliced 1/4 inch thick
- 2 Cup cream
- 1 Tablespoon minced sage
- 1 Cup shredded Gruyere or other hearty Swiss cheese, divided

Directions:
1. Supply your smoker with wood pellets and follow the start-up procedure. Preheat the grill, with the lid closed, to 400° F.

2. Butter a 9x13 baking dish with 1 tablespoon of the softened butter. In a medium frying pan over medium heat, melt the remaining butter. Add the leeks and a generous pinch of salt and pepper and cook, stirring often until softened, about 5 minutes.

3. Remove from the heat and allow to cool. Place the potato and celery root slices into a large mixing bowl. Add the cream, leek mixture, minced sage, 1 teaspoon salt, 1/2 teaspoon pepper and 1 cup cheese. Stir gently to coat.

4. Arrange a layer of potato and celery root slices so they're slightly overlapping in the prepared baking dish. Repeat two more times so there are three layers of potatoes. Pour remaining cream from the bowl over the gratin, then sprinkle the top with the remaining cup of cheese.

5. Cover the dish loosely with foil and bake on the grill for 45 minutes. Remove the foil and continue baking until the top is golden and bubbly and the potatoes are tender when pierced, about 30 to 45 minutes longer. Let stand for 10 minutes before serving. Enjoy!

Baked Irish Creme Cake

Servings: 4
Cooking Time: 60 Minutes

Ingredients:
- 1 Cup Pecans, pieces
- 1 Yellow Cake Mix, Boxed
- 1 Vanilla Pudding Mix, Instant Package (3.4oz)
- 4 Large eggs
- 1/2 Cup water
- 1/2 Cup vegetable oil
- 1 Cup Irish Cream Liquor
- 1/2 Cup butter
- 1 Cup sugar

Directions:
1. Grease and flour a 10" (25 cm) Bundt pan. Sprinkle pecans along the bottom.

2. In a large bowl, with a mixer, combine yellow cake mix, pudding mix, eggs, water, oil, and Irish Cream liquor. Pour batter over nuts in the pan.

3.   Supply your smoker with wood pellets and follow the start-up procedure. Preheat the grill, with the lid closed, to 325° F.

4.   Place Bundt pan on the Traeger and bake for 1 hour, or until a toothpick comes out clean. Remove from heat, cool for 10 minutes. Grill: 325 ℉

5.   While the cake is cooling, combine the butter, water and sugar and bring to a boil. Boil for 5 minutes, stirring constantly. Remove from heat and add Irish cream liquor.

6.   Use a bamboo skewer to poke holes in the cooled cake. Spoon glaze over the cake. Allow cake to absorb the glaze. Enjoy!

Chocolate Lava Cake With Smoked Whipped Cream

Servings: 4
Cooking Time: 45 Minutes

Ingredients:
- 1 Pint heavy whipping cream
- 9 Tablespoon Butter
- 220 G Semisweet Chocolate
- 1 1/4 Cup powdered sugar
- 2 Large eggs
- 2 egg yolk
- 6 Tablespoon flour
- 1 Tablespoon Bourbon Vanilla
- Powdered Sugar
- cocoa powder

Directions:

1.   Supply your smoker with wood pellets and follow the start-up procedure. Preheat the grill, with the lid closed, to 180° F.

2.   For the Smoked Whipped Cream: Add cream to a shallow, aluminum baking pan. Place the pan on the grill and smoke for 30 minutes.

3.   Pour the smoked cream into a large mixing bowl and refrigerate for later use. Grill: 180 ℉

4.   Increase the grill temperature to 375°F and preheat. Grill: 375 ℉

5.   Brush 4 small soufflé cups with 1 tablespoon melted butter.

6.   Melt the chocolate and remaining butter in a heatproof bowl over simmering water, stir until smooth.

7.   Stir in powdered sugar. Add eggs and egg yolks, stirring continuously. Whisk in flour until blended completely.

8.   Pour batter into the prepared soufflé cups. Place them on the Traeger and bake for 13-14 minutes, or until the sides are set. Grill: 375 ℉

9.   For the Whipped Cream: Remove the chilled smoked cream from the refrigerator, add the bourbon vanilla and whip until airy.

10. Add confectioners sugar and continue whipping until whipped cream forms stiff peaks.

11. Dust lava cakes with confectioners sugar and cocoa, top with a dollop of smoke-infused whipped cream. Enjoy!

Eggs Ham Benedict

Servings: 6
Cooking Time: 15 Minutes

Ingredients:
- 1 Biscuit Dough, Tube
- 6 Egg
- 16 Ham, Sliced
- 1 Packet Hollandaise Sauce, Package

Directions:

1.   Supply your smoker with wood pellets and follow the start-up procedure. Preheat the grill, with the lid closed, to 350° F.

2. Grease a muffin tin and crack an egg in each cup. Place on the grate of the for about 10 minutes or until the whites are fully cooked.

3. At the same time, place your biscuit dough on a greased pan. Follow the directions on the packaging but bake on the . Place 2 slices of ham per biscuit on the pan as well.

4. While the ham, eggs, and biscuits are cooking, prepare the Hollandaise Sauce according to the directions on the packet.

5. When everything is fully cooked, cut a biscuit in half, and stack one or two slices of ham, 1 egg and a dollop of Hollandaise sauce. Repeat for each half biscuit. Serve with fresh fruit.

Baked Chocolate Brownie Cookies With Egg Nog

Servings: 6
Cooking Time: 12 Minutes

Ingredients:
- 16 Ounce Bar bittersweet chocolate, finely chopped
- 4 Tablespoon unsalted butter, room temperature
- 4 eggs
- 1 1/3 Cup granulated sugar
- 1 Teaspoon vanilla extract
- 1 1/2 Cup all-purpose flour
- 1/2 Teaspoon baking powder
- 1 Cup semisweet chocolate chips

Directions:
1. Supply your smoker with wood pellets and follow the start-up procedure. Preheat the grill, with the lid closed, to 350° F.

2. Line two baking sheets with parchment paper.

3. Put the finely chopped chocolate and butter in a heatproof bowl and set over a saucepan of barely simmering water; stir occasionally until chocolate is completely melted and smooth. Set aside and allow to cool to room temperature.

4. Whisk together eggs, sugar and vanilla extract in a medium bowl. Set aside.

5. Sift together the flour and baking powder in a small bowl. Add the melted chocolate mixture to the egg mixture and stir with a rubber spatula until completely combined.

6. Add the flour mixture in three batches, folding gently into the batter with a spatula. Once all of the flour has been incorporated, stir in the chocolate chips.

7. Scoop 1-1/2 tablespoons of dough onto prepared baking sheets. Bake for 10 to 12 minutes or until they are firm on the outside. Do not over bake. Grill:350° F

8. Leave to cool completely on the baking sheets. Enjoy!

Smoked Lemon Tea

Servings: 6 - 8
Cooking Time: 60 Minutes

Ingredients:
- 8 Black Tea Bags
- 4 Cups Boiling Water
- 2 Cups Ice
- 8 Lemons
- 2 Cups Sugar
- 2 Cups Water

Directions:
1. Place the tea bags in a heat-safe pitcher. Bring 4 Cups of water to a boil and pour over tea bags. Let steep for 5-10 minutes. Remove tea bags and set pitcher aside to cool.

2. Turn on your grill and set to smoke mode. Combine 2 cups of sugar and 2 cups water in a

small aluminum pan. Smoke for about 45 minutes, stirring occasionally, or until the mixture reduces to a thick, simple syrup. Remove from the grill and let it cool.

3. Supply your smoker with wood pellets and follow the start-up procedure. Preheat the grill, with the lid closed, to 450° F. If using a charcoal or gas grill, set heat to high.

4. Cut the lemons in half and sear over the flame broiler until charred, about 7 minutes. Remove from grill and set aside to cool.

5. Juice the lemons into a medium bowl. Pour lemon juice through a metal strainer into the tea pitcher to remove seeds and pulp.

6. Pour the cooled simple syrup into pitcher and stir until fully incorporated with tea and lemons. Add 2 cups of ice and refrigerate until serving.

Smoked Lemon Cheesecake

Servings: 16
Cooking Time: 130 Minutes

Ingredients:
- For the crust
- Vegetable oil, for oiling the pan
- 12 ounces gingersnaps (about 36) or chocolate icebox cookies (about 36)
- 3 tablespoons light brown sugar
- 8 tablespoons (1 stick) unsalted butter, melted
- For the filling
- 4 packages (8 ounces each) cream cheese, at room temperature
- 1 cup firmly packed light brown sugar
- 2 teaspoons pure vanilla extract
- 2 teaspoons finely grated lemon zest
- 1 tablespoon fresh lemon juice
- 2 tablespoons (1/4 stick) unsalted butter, melted

- 5 large eggs
- Burnt Sugar Sauce (recipes follows, optional)

Directions:

1. Supply your smoker with wood pellets and follow the start-up procedure. Preheat the grill, with the lid closed, to 400° F. Lightly oil the springform pan with vegetable oil and wrap a sheet of aluminum foil around the outside.

2. Make the crust: Break the cookies into pieces and grind with the brown sugar to a fine powder in a food processor. You'll want about 1 3/4 cups of crumbs. Add the melted butter and run the processor in short bursts to obtain a crumbly dough. Press the mixture evenly across the bottom and halfway up the sides of the springform pan. Indirect-grill or bake the crust until lightly browned, 5 to 8 minutes. Transfer the pan to a wire rack and let cool.

3. Make the filling: Wipe out the food processor bowl. Add the cream cheese, brown sugar, vanilla, lemon zest, lemon juice, and butter, and process until smooth. Work in the eggs one by one, processing until smooth after each addition. (You can also use a stand mixer, beating the cream cheese mixture until smooth and beating in the eggs one at a time.) Pour the filling into the crust. Gently tap the pan on the countertop a few times to knock out any air bubbles.

4. Supply your smoker with wood pellets and follow the start-up procedure. Preheat the grill, with the lid closed, to 225 °F-250 °F.

5. Place the cheesecake in the smoker. Smoke until the top is bronzed with smoke and the filling is set, 1 1/2 to 2 hours. To test for doneness, gently poke the side of the pan—the filling will jiggle, not ripple. Alternatively, insert a

slender metal skewer in the center of the cake; it should come out clean.

6. Transfer the cheesecake in its pan to a wire rack to cool to room temperature. Refrigerate until serving; the cheesecake can be made up to 8 hours ahead. Run a slender knife around the inside of the springform pan. Unclasp and remove the ring. (You'll serve the cheesecake off the bottom of the pan.) Let the cheesecake warm slightly at room temperature before serving.

7. If serving with the sauce, pour some of it over the cheesecake and the rest into a pitcher. Cut into wedges and pass the remaining sauce.

Chicken Pot Pie

Servings: 6
Cooking Time: 60 Minutes

Ingredients:
- 2 Chicken, Boneless/Skinless
- 1 Cream Of Chicken Soup, Can
- 1 Tsp Curry Powder
- 1/2 Cup Mayo
- 1 1/2 Cups Mixed Frozen Vegetables
- 1 Onion, Sliced
- 2 Frozen Pie Shell, Deep
- 1/2 Cup Sour Cream

Directions:
1. Supply your smoker with wood pellets and follow the start-up procedure. Preheat the grill, with the lid closed, to 425° F.
2. Cut the onion in half and place on the grates of the grill. If you"re using fresh chicken breasts, barbecue the chicken at the same time as the onions. The chicken is fully cooked when the internal temperature reached 170F. While the onion and chicken are cooking, prepare the pie crust by putting one crust in a pie plate. When the chicken and onions are done, shred chicken and chop onion into small pieces and place in the prepared pie plate along with the mixed vegetables.

3. Combine cream of chicken soup, mayo, sour cream, and curry powder in a bowl. Pour into the pie crust with the chicken and mix to combine. Wet the sides of the bottom crust with a small amount of water and top with the second pie crust. Push gently along the sides of the crust to seal the two pie crusts together.

4. Place in the and bake for 40 minutes, or until the crust is golden brown. Serve hot.

Cherry Ice Cream Cobbler

Servings: 8
Cooking Time: 45 Minutes

Ingredients:
- 1 Tsp Baking Powder
- 3 Tbsp Butter, Melted
- 1 Cup Flour
- Ice Cream, Prepared
- 1/4 Tsp Salt
- 3/4 Cup Sugar
- 1/2 Cup Milk

Directions:
1. Supply your smoker with wood pellets and follow the start-up procedure. Preheat the grill, with the lid closed, to 350° F.
2. In a bowl, combine flour, sugar, baking powder, salt and mix to incorporate. Stir in butter and milk and mix until combined. In a cast iron pan, dump in cherry pie filling and pile on the prepared topping to cover.
3. Place in your Grill and bake for about 45 minutes, or until the topping is golden brown.
4. Let cool for a couple minutes and serve with ice cream.

Vanilla Cheesecake Skillet Brownie

Servings: 2
Cooking Time: 30 Minutes

Ingredients:

➢ 1 Box Brownie Mix
➢ 1 Package Cream Cheese
➢ 2 Egg
➢ 1/2 Cup Oil
➢ 1 Can Pie Filling, Blueberry
➢ 1/2 Cup Sugar
➢ 1 Tsp Vanilla
➢ 1/4 Cup Water, Warm

Directions:

1. Combine all brownie ingredients and mix. In a separate bowl, combine cream cheese, sugar, egg and vanilla and mix until smooth. Grease skillets and pour in brownie batter. Top with cheesecake and cherry pie filling, using a knife to blend to give it that marbled look.

2. Supply your smoker with wood pellets and follow the start-up procedure. Preheat the grill, with the lid closed, to 350°F and bake for about 30 minutes.

3. Let cool for about 10 minutes and enjoy!

Grilled Apple Pie

Servings: 4
Cooking Time: 40 Minutes

Ingredients:

➢ 5 Whole Apples
➢ 1/4 Cup sugar
➢ 1 Tablespoon cornstarch
➢ 1 Whole refrigerated pie crust
➢ 1/4 Cup Peach, preserves

Directions:

1. Supply your smoker with wood pellets and follow the start-up procedure. Preheat the grill, with the lid closed, to 375° F.In a medium bowl, mix the apples, sugar, and cornstarch; set aside.

2. Unroll pie crust. Place in ungreased pie pan. With the back of a spoon, spread preserves evenly on crust. Arrange the apple slices in an even layer in the pie pan. Slightly fold crust over filling.

3. Place a baking sheet upside down on the grill grate to make an elevated surface. Put the pan with pie on top so it is elevated off grill. (This will help prevent the bottom from overcooking.) Cook the pie for 30 to 40 minutes or until crust is golden brown, the filling is bubbly. Grill: 375 °F

4. Remove from grill; cool 10 minutes before serving. Enjoy! *Cook times will vary depending on set and ambient temperatures.

Ultimate Baked Garlic Bread

Servings: 4
Cooking Time: 20 Minutes

Ingredients:

➢ 1 baguette
➢ 1/2 Cup softened butter
➢ 1/2 Cup mayonnaise
➢ 4 Tablespoon chopped Italian parsley
➢ 6 Clove garlic, minced
➢ salt
➢ chile flakes
➢ 1 Cup mozzarella cheese
➢ 1/2 Cup Parmesan cheese

Directions:

1. Supply your smoker with wood pellets and follow the start-up procedure. Preheat the grill, with the lid closed, to 375° F.

2. Lay baguette on a cutting board and cut it in half lengthwise.

3. In a bowl, add butter, mayonnaise, parsley, garlic, salt and chile flakes. Mix well.

4. Spread butter mixture on baguette halves and top with mozzarella and Parmesan cheese.

5. Place baguette on the grill (if you like the bread crisp, do not use foil and if you like it soft, wrap with foil). Grill for approximately 15 to 25 minutes. Serve warm. Enjoy! Grill: 375 ℉

Blueberry Bread Pudding

Servings: 4
Cooking Time: 60 Minutes

Ingredients:

- 5 eggs
- 3 Cup sugar
- 2 1/2 Cup milk
- 1 1/2 Teaspoon vanilla
- 1 Teaspoon cinnamon
- 1 Pinch salt
- 5 Cup Bread
- 3 Cup blueberries

Directions:

1. Beat the eggs in a large mixing bowl. Whisk in the sugar, milk, vanilla, cinnamon, and salt.

2. In another large bowl, combine the bread and 2 cups (200 g) of the blueberries.

3. Pour the egg mixture over the bread-blueberry mixture and let sit for 30 minutes. Meanwhile, place muffin liners in a muffin tin.

4. Supply your smoker with wood pellets and follow the start-up procedure. Preheat the grill, with the lid open.

5. Spoon the bread-blueberry mixture into the prepared cups; evenly top each with the remaining cup of blueberries, pressing them gently into the pudding with the back of a spoon.

6. Dust the top with sugar.

7. Arrange the pan directly on the grill grate and smoke for 30 minutes. Grill:180℉

8. Increase the temperature to 350F (180 C), and bake until the pudding is set and golden brown on top, about 25 minutes. Grill:350℉

9. Let cool slightly, then sift powdered sugar on top. Serve warm with sweetened whipped cream or vanilla ice cream, if desired.

Sopapilla Cheesecake By Doug Scheiding

Servings: 8
Cooking Time: 45 Minutes

Ingredients:

- 2 Tablespoon softened butter
- 24 Ounce cream cheese
- 2 Cup granulated sugar, divided
- 2 Teaspoon vanilla
- 2 Can Pillsbury Butter Flake Crescent Rolls
- 1/2 Cup butter, melted
- cinnamon

Directions:

1. Coat a 9x13 inch baking dish with 2 tablespoons softened butter and set aside.

2. Supply your smoker with wood pellets and follow the start-up procedure. Preheat the grill, with the lid closed, to 350° F.

3. In a mixer, combine cream cheese, 1 to 1-1/2 cups of sugar and vanilla. Mix for 60 to 90 seconds on high with paddle attachment.

4. Take crescents out of the refrigerator. Open one can and place into the buttered 9x13 inch rectangular metal pan or glass dish. Make sure to fill in the gaps in this bottom layer of crescents.

5. Put the cream cheese mixture on the top of the crescent layer using a spatula to make it level.

6. Open the second can of crescents and put on top of the cream cheese layer, again filling in the gaps in the crescents to cover middle.

7. Pour 1/2 cup of melted butter on the top of the last layer of crescent. Start on sides first then middle.

8. Then sprinkle 1/4 cup to 1/2 cup of sugar over the entire pan followed by a light, even dusting of cinnamon.

9. Place pan directly on the grill grate and bake for 40 to 50 minutes until top is brown and starting to get crusty. Grill: 350 ˚F

10. Remove from grill and let cool 5 to 10 minutes. This allows the cheesecake to set which makes portioning easier. This dessert can be served warm or cold. Enjoy!

Pizza Bites

Servings: 6
Cooking Time: 20 Minutes

Ingredients:

➢ 4 1/2 Cup Bread Flour
➢ 1 1/2 Tablespoon sugar
➢ 2 Teaspoon Instant Yeast
➢ 2 Teaspoon kosher salt
➢ 3 Tablespoon extra-virgin olive oil
➢ 15 Fluid Ounce Water, Lukewarm
➢ 8 Ounce Pepperoni, sliced
➢ 1 Cup pizza sauce
➢ 1 Cup mozzarella cheese
➢ 1 Whole egg, for egg wash
➢ 1 As Needed salt

Directions:

1. For the Pizza Dough: Combine flour, sugar, salt, and yeast in food processor. Pulse 3 to 4 times until incorporated evenly. Add olive oil and water. Run food processor until mixture forms ball that rides around the bowl above the blade, about 15 seconds. Continue processing 15 seconds longer.

2. Transfer dough ball to lightly floured surface and knead once or twice by hand until smooth ball is formed. Divide dough into three even parts and place each into a 1 gallon zip top bag. Place in refrigerator and allow to rise at least one day.

3. At least two hours before baking, remove dough from refrigerator and shape into balls by gathering dough towards bottom and pinching shut. Flour well and place each one in a separate medium mixing bowl. Cover tightly with plastic wrap and allow to rise at warm room temperature until roughly doubled in volume.

4. When ready to cook, set the grill temperature to 350°F and preheat, lid closed for 15 minutes.

5. After the first rise remove the dough from the fridge and let come to room temperature. Roll dough on a flat surface. Cut dough into long strips 3" wide by 18" long.

6. Slice pepperoni into strips.

7. In a medium bowl combine the pizza sauce, mozzarella and pepperoni.

8. Spoon 1 TBSP of the pizza filling onto the pizza dough every two inches, about halfway down the length of the dough. Dip a pastry brush into the egg wash and brush around pizza filling. Fold the half side of the dough (without the pizza filling) over the other the half that contains the pizza filling.

9. Press down between each pizza bite slightly with your fingers. With a ravioli or pizza cutter, cut around each filling- creating a rectangle shape and sealing the crust in.

10. Transfer each pizza bite onto a parchment lined cookie sheet. Cover with a kitchen towel and let them rise for 30 minutes.

11. When ready to cook, preheat the grill to 350 ⯑ ℉ with the lid closed for 10-15 minutes.

12. Brush the bites with remaining egg wash, sprinkle with salt and place directly on the sheet tray. Bake 10-15 minutes until the exterior is golden brown.

13. Remove from grill and transfer to a serving dish. Serve with extra pizza sauce for dipping and enjoy!

Delicious Peanut Butter Cookies

Servings: 24
Cooking Time: 15 Minutes

Ingredients:
- 1 Egg
- 1 Cup Peanut Butter
- 1 Cup Sugar

Directions:
1. Supply your smoker with wood pellets and follow the start-up procedure. Preheat the grill, with the lid closed, to High heat.

2. Combine all ingredients in a bowl. Drop tablespoon amounts of dough on a prepared baking sheet and bake in your Grill for 15-20 minutes. Allow cookies to cool for 5 minutes on the baking sheet before you enjoy!

Focaccia

Servings: 6
Cooking Time: 40 Minutes

Ingredients:
- 1 Cup warm water (110°F to 115°F)
- 1/2 Ounce Yeast, active
- 1 Teaspoon sugar
- 2 1/2 Cup flour
- 1 Teaspoon salt
- 1/4 Cup extra-virgin olive oil
- 1 1/2 Teaspoon Italian herbs, dried
- 1/8 Teaspoon red pepper flakes
- As Needed coarse sea salt

Directions:
1. Measure the water in a glass-measuring cup. Stir in the yeast and sugar. Let rest for in a warm place. After 5 to 10 minutes, the mixture should be foamy, indicating the yeast is "alive." If it does not foam, discard it and start again.

2. Pour the water/yeast mixture in the bowl of a food processor. Add 1 cup of the flour as well as the salt and 1/4 cup of olive oil. Pulse several times to blend. Add the remaining flour, Italian herbs, and hot pepper flakes.

3. Process the dough until it's smooth and elastic and pulls away from the sides of the bowl, adding small amounts of flour or water through the feed tube if the dough is respectively too wet or too dry.

4. Let the dough rise in the covered food processor bowl in a warm place until doubled in bulk, about 1 hour5. Remove the dough from the food processor (it will deflate) and turn onto a lightly floured surface.

5. Oil two 8- to 9-inch round cake pans generously with olive oil. (Just pour a couple of glugs in and tilt the pan to spread the oil.) Divide the dough into two equal pieces, shape into disks, and put one in each prepared cake pan.

6. Oil the top of each disk with olive oil and dimple the dough with your fingertips. Sprinkle lightly with coarse salt, and if desired, additional dried Italian herbs.

7. Cover the focaccia dough with plastic wrap and let the dough rise in a warm place, about 45 minutes to an hour.

8. When ready to cook, start the smoker grill and set the temperature to 400F and preheat, lid closed, for 10 to 15 minutes.

9. Put the pans with the focaccia dough directly on the grill grate. Bake until the focaccia breads are light golden in color and baked through, 35 to 40 minutes, rotating the pans halfway through the baking time.

10. Let cool slightly before removing from the pans. Cut into wedges for serving.

Lemon Chicken, Broccoli, String Beans Foil Packs

Servings: 4

Cooking Time: 20 Minutes

Ingredients:

➢ 2 Cups Broccoli

➢ 3 Tbsp Butter, Melted

➢ 4 Chicken, Boneless/Skinless

➢ 1 Garlic, Minced

➢ 1 1/2 Tsp Italian Seasoning, Dried

➢ 1 Lemon, Sliced

➢ Pepper

➢ Salt

➢ 1 Cup String Beans

Directions:

1. Supply your smoker with wood pellets and follow the start-up procedure. Preheat the grill, with the lid closed, to 450° F.

2. Lay four 12 x 12 inch pieces of foil out on a flat surface, then place one chicken breast in the middle of each foil.

3. Divide the broccoli and string beans between the four foil packs. Thinly slice the lemon, split

them between each foil pack, and place the slices on, in and around the chicken and vegetables.

4. Mix the butter, garlic, juice of the remaining lemon, and Italian seasoning together, and then brush over the chicken and vegetables. Sprinkle with salt and pepper to taste.

5. Fold the foil over the chicken and vegetables to close the pack, and pinch the ends together so the pack will remain closed.

6. Grill for 7-9 minutes on each side. Turn off grill, remove the foil packets, and serve immediately.

Basil Margherita Pizza

Servings: 6

Cooking Time: 25 Minutes

Ingredients:

➢ Basil, Chopped

➢ 2 Cups Flour, All-Purpose

➢ Mozzarella Cheese, Sliced Rounds

➢ 1 Cup Pizza Sauce

➢ 1 Teaspoon Salt

➢ 1 Teaspoon Sugar

➢ 1 Tomato, Sliced

➢ 1 Cup Water, Warm

➢ 1 Teaspoon Yeast, Instant

Directions:

1. Combine the water, yeast, and sugar in a small bowl and let sit for about 5 minutes.

2. In a large bowl, stir together the flour and salt. Pour in the yeast mixture and mix until a soft dough forms. Knead for about 2 minutes. Place in an oiled bowl and cover with a cloth. Let the dough sit and rise for about 45 minutes or until the dough has doubled in size.

3. Roll out on a flat, floured surface (or on a pizza stone) until you''ve reached your desired shape and thickness.

4. Supply your smoker with wood pellets and follow the start-up procedure. Preheat the grill, with the lid closed, to 350° F.

5. On the rolled out dough, pour on the pizza sauce, cheese, and then tomatoes and basil. Place in your Grill and bake for about 25 minutes, or until the cheese is melted and slightly golden brown.

Double Vanilla Chocolate Cake

Servings: 12
Cooking Time: 40 Minutes

Ingredients:

- 1 1/2 Tsp Baking Soda
- 1/2 Cup Butter, Melted
- 1 Cup Buttermilk, Low Fat
- 1 Jar Chocolate Icing, Prepared
- 3/4 Cup Cocoa, Powder
- 1 Cup Coffee, Hot
- 2 Large Egg
- 1 3/4 Cups Flour, All-Purpose
- 3/4 Tsp Salt
- 2 Cups Sugar
- 1 Tbsp Vanilla

Directions:

1. Supply your smoker with wood pellets and follow the start-up procedure. Preheat the grill, with the lid closed, to 350° F.

2. Stir together flour, sugar, cocoa, baking soda and salt in a large bowl. Combine eggs, buttermilk, butter and coffee and mix until smooth. Add in hot coffee and stir until combined and the dough is runny.

3. Pour the batter into two prepared baking pans and bake on the top rack of your for 40 minutes, turning the pans 180 degrees halfway through.

4. Allow to cool and then frost with chocolate icing.

Zucchini Bread

Servings: 6
Cooking Time: 50 Minutes

Ingredients:

- 1 Cup Walnuts, Chopped
- 2 Large zucchini
- 1 Teaspoon salt
- 1 Teaspoon ground cinnamon
- 1/4 Teaspoon ground cloves
- 1/4 Teaspoon baking powder
- 3 Cup all-purpose flour
- 1 eggs
- 2 Cup sugar
- 1/2 Cup vegetable oil
- 1/2 Cup Yogurt
- 1 1/2 Teaspoon vanilla extract

Directions:

1. Grease and flour two 9- by 5-inch bread pans, preferably nonstick.

2. When ready to cook, set the temperature to 350℉ and preheat, lid closed for 15 minutes.

3. Spread the walnuts on a pie plate and toast for 10 minutes, stirring once. Let cool, then coarsely chop. Set aside.

4. Trim the ends off the zucchini, then coarsely grate into a colander set over the sink on a box grater (or use the shredding disk on a food processor). You'll need 2 cups.

5. Sprinkle with the salt and let drain for 30 minutes. Press on the zucchini with paper towels to expel excess water.

6. Sift the flour, baking powder, cinnamon, and cloves in a mixing bowl or on a large sheet of parchment or wax paper.

7. Combine the eggs, sugar, oil, yogurt, and vanilla in a large mixing bowl and mix on medium speed. (You can mix the batter by hand, if desired.) Add half the dry ingredients and mix on low speed; add the remaining dry ingredients and mix until just combined.

8. Stir in the walnuts and zucchini by hand.

9. Divide the batter between the prepared baking pans.

10. Arrange the pans directly on the grill grate and bake for 50 minutes, or until a bamboo skewer inserted in the center of the breads comes out clean.

11. Transfer to a wire rack and let cool for 10 minutes, then remove the breads from the pans. For best results, let the breads cool completely before slicing.

Donut Bread Pudding

Servings: 8
Cooking Time: 40 Minutes

Ingredients:
- 16 Cake Donuts
- 1/2 Cup Raisins, seedless
- 5 eggs
- 3/4 Cup sugar
- 2 Cup heavy cream
- 2 Teaspoon vanilla extract
- 1 Teaspoon ground cinnamon
- 3/4 Cup Butter, melted, cooled slightly
- Ice Cream

Directions:
1. Lightly butter a 9- by 13-inch baking pan. Layer the donuts in an even thickness in the pan.

Distribute the raisins over the top, if using. Drizzle evenly with the butter.

2. Make the custard: In a medium bowl, whisk together the sugar, eggs, cream, vanilla, and cinnamon. Whisk in the butter. Pour over the donuts. Let sit for 10 to 15 minutes, periodically pushing the donuts down into the custard. Cover with foil.

3. Supply your smoker with wood pellets and follow the start-up procedure. Preheat the grill, with the lid closed, to 350° F.

4. Bake the bread pudding for 30 to 40 minutes, or until the custard is set. Remove the foil and continue to bake for 10 additional minutes to lightly brown the top. Grill: 350 ˚F

5. Let cool slightly before cutting into squares. Drizzle with melted ice cream, if desired. Enjoy!

Smoked Sweet Beer Bread

Servings: 6
Cooking Time: 60 Minutes

Ingredients:
- 3 cups all-purpose flour, sifted
- 2 tbsp. sugar
- 1 tbsp. baking powder
- 1 tsp. salt
- 1 (12 oz) can or bottle beer (not too dark or bitter)
- 2 tbsp. honey or agave, warmed
- 6 tbsp. butter, melted

Directions:
1. Supply your smoker with wood pellets and follow the start-up procedure. Preheat the grill, with the lid closed, to 350° F.

2. Lightly grease a 9 ×5 inch loaf pan.

3. In a large mixing bowl, put in the flour, sugar, baking powder, and salt. Whisk to combine and

aerate, using a wire whisk. Add the beer and honey and stir with a wooden spoon until the batter is properly mixed (Do not over-mix).

4. Pour half of the melted butter into the prepared loaf pan and pour in the batter. Pour the remaining butter over the top of the loaf.

5. Place the loaf pan on the grill grate and bake for 50 to 60 minutes or until the bread is golden brown.

6. Allow the loaf to cool slightly in the pan before removing it from the pan. Leftovers make great toast.

Baked Chocolate Coconut Brownies

Servings: 4

Cooking Time: 25 Minutes

Ingredients:
- 1/2 Cup gluten-free or all-purpose flour, such as Bob's Red Mill
- 1/4 Cup unsweetened alkalized cocoa powder
- 1/2 Teaspoon sea salt
- 4 Ounce semisweet chocolate, coarsely chopped
- 3/4 Cup unrefined coconut oil
- 1 Cup raw cane sugar
- 4 eggs
- 1 Teaspoon vanilla extract
- 4 Ounce semisweet chocolate chips, optional

Directions:

1. Supply your smoker with wood pellets and follow the start-up procedure. Preheat the grill, with the lid closed, to 350° F.

2. Grease a 9x9 inch baking pan and line with parchment paper.

3. Combine the flour, cocoa powder and salt in a medium bowl. Set aside.

4. In a double boiler or microwave, melt the chopped chocolate and coconut oil. Let cool slightly.

5. Add the sugar, eggs and vanilla. Whisking until well combined.

6. Whisk in the flour mixture and fold in the chocolate chips. Pour into the prepared pan.

7. Place on the grill and bake until a toothpick inserted in the center of the brownies comes out clean, about 20 to 25 minutes. This will yield a somewhat gooey brownie. Continue to bake for 5 to 10 minutes if you prefer a drier brownie. Grill: 350 °F

8. Let the brownies cool completely, then cut into squares. Store in an airtight container at room temperature for up to 3 days. Enjoy!

SEAFOOD RECIPES

Smoked Trout

Servings: 6
Cooking Time: 120 Minutes

Ingredients:
- 8 rainbow trout fillets
- 1 Gallon water
- 1/4 Cup salt
- 1/2 Cup brown sugar
- 1 Tablespoon black pepper
- 2 Tablespoon soy sauce

Directions:
1. Clean the fresh fish and butterfly them.
2. For the Brine: Combine one gallon water, brown sugar, soy sauce, salt and pepper and stir until salt and sugar are dissolved. Brine the trout in the refrigerator for 60 minutes.
3. Supply your smoker with wood pellets and follow the start-up procedure. Preheat the grill, with the lid closed, to 225° F.
4. Remove the fish from the brine and pat dry. Place fish directly on grill grate for 1-1/2 to 2 hours, depending on the thickness of the trout. Fish is done when it turns opaque and starts to flake. Serve hot or cold. Enjoy! Grill: 225 ˚F
5. Fish is done when it turns opaque and starts to flake. Serve hot or cold. Enjoy!

Lime Mahi Mahi Fillets

Servings: 4
Cooking Time: 8 Minutes

Ingredients:
- 3/4 cup extra-virgin olive oil
- 1 clove garlic, minced
- 1/8 teaspoon ground black pepper
- 1/2 teaspoon cayenne pepper
- 2 tablespoons dill weed.
- 1 pinch salt
- 2 tablespoons lime juice
- 1/8 teaspoon grated lime peel
- 2 (4 ounce) mahi mahi fillets

Directions:
1. Supply your smoker with wood pellets and follow the start-up procedure. Preheat the grill, with the lid closed, to 325° F.
2. Lightly oil the grate.
3. Combine in a bowl the extra-virgin olive oil, minced garlic, black pepper, cayenne pepper, salt, lime juice, and grated lime zest.
4. Wisk to prepare the marinade.
5. Place the mahi mahi fillets in the marinade and turn to coat.
6. Allow to marinate at least 15 minutes.
7. Cook on preheated grill until fish flakes easily with a fork and is lightly browned (Typically 3 to 4 minutes per side).
8. Garnish with the twists of lime zest to serve.

Spicy Crab Poppers

Servings: 8
Cooking Time: 30 Minutes

Ingredients:
- 18 Whole jalapeño
- 8 Ounce cream cheese, softened
- 1 Cup Canned Corn, drained
- 1/2 Cup Crab meat, lump
- 1 1/4 Teaspoon Old Bay Seasoning
- 2 Scallions, minced

Directions:

1. Cut each jalapeño in half lengthwise through the stem and remove the ribs and seeds.

2. Filling: In a mixing bowl, combine the cream cheese, corn, crab meat, scallions, and Old Bay Seasoning and stir until blended. Stir in the scallions. Spoon the filling into the jalapeño halves, mounding it slightly.

3. Arrange the poppers on a baking sheet covered with foil or parchment paper.

4. Supply your smoker with wood pellets and follow the start-up procedure. Preheat the grill, with the lid closed, to 350° F.

5. Roast the jalapeños for 25 to 30 minutes, or until the peppers have softened and the filling is hot and bubbling.

6. Let cool slightly before serving. Enjoy!

Planked Trout With Fennel, Bacon & Orange

Servings: 4
Cooking Time: 40minutes

Ingredients:
- 4 whole trout, each about 14 to 16oz (400 to 450g), cleaned and gutted, fins removed
- coarse salt
- freshly ground black pepper
- for the filling
- 1 large navel orange
- 4 slices of thick-cut bacon, diced
- 1 large fennel bulb, trimmed, halved, decored, and diced, green fronds reserved
- 4oz (110g) baby spinach, about 6 cups
- coarse salt
- freshly ground black pepper

Directions:
1. Supply your smoker with wood pellets and follow the start-up procedure. Preheat the grill, with the lid closed, to 450° F. Place 4 cedar planks on the grate and allow them to singe slightly on both sides. Remove them from the grill and place them on a heatproof surface to cool.

2. Lower the temperature to 300°F (149°C).

3. Slice 4 thin rounds from the center of the orange and then slice each in half for 8 pieces total. Zest the remainder of the orange and set aside.

4. In a cold skillet on the stovetop over medium heat, sauté the bacon, until the fat has rendered and the bacon is golden brown, about 6 to 8 minutes, stirring frequently. Use a slotted spoon to transfer the bacon to paper towels to drain. Add the fennel to the fat in the skillet and cook until tender crisp, about 5 minutes. Add the spinach and stir until it wilts, about 1 to 2 minutes. Squeeze the juice of one of the reserved orange ends over the mixture. Add the drained bacon. Season with salt and pepper and then stir. Remove the skillet from the stovetop and set aside.

5. Rinse each trout inside and out under cold running water and pat dry with paper towels. Place three 12-inch (30.5cm) pieces of butcher's twine on each plank and place a trout on top. Season the inside of each fish with salt and pepper. Place two half-rounds of orange in each belly, rind side facing out. Top with some of the filling. Tie the trout with the butcher's twine and trim any ends. Repeat with the remaining trout.

6. Place the planks on the grate and cook the trout until they're cooked through, about 30 to 40 minutes.

7. Remove the planks from the grill and remove the twine. Top each trout with a few curls of orange zest and some reserved fennel fronds. Serve the trout on the planks.

Florentine Shrimp Al Cartoccio

Servings: 4

Cooking Time: 13 Minutes

Ingredients:

- 6 tbsp unsalted butter, melted
- ½ cup heavy whipping cream
- ½ cup grated Parmesan cheese
- 2 garlic cloves, peeled and minced
- 1 cup thinly sliced button mushrooms, cleaned and destemmed
- 1 cup baby spinach leaves
- 2 tbsp chopped sun-dried, oil-packed tomatoes
- ½ tsp dried oregano
- ½ tsp dried basil
- ½ tsp crushed red pepper flakes, plus more
- ½ tsp coarse salt
- ½ tsp freshly ground black pepper
- 20 to 24 jumbo shrimp, about 1lb (450g) total, peeled and deveined
- sprigs of fresh rosemary, basil, thyme, or oregano

Directions:

1. Supply your smoker with wood pellets and follow the start-up procedure. Preheat the grill, with the lid closed, to 400° F.

2. In a large bowl, combine the butter and whipping cream. Stir in the Parmesan, garlic, mushrooms, spinach, tomatoes, oregano, basil, red pepper flakes, and salt and pepper. Add the shrimp and stir gently to coat.

3. Place four 12-inch (30.5cm) sheets of wide heavy-duty aluminum foil on a workspace and pull up the sides. Divide the shrimp mixture evenly between the sheets of foil. Roll and crimp the top and sides of the foil to create sealed packages.

4. Place the packets seam side up on the grate and grill until the shrimp are cooked through, about 10 to 13 minutes. (You can carefully open one package to check on the shrimp.)

5. Transfer the packets to plates. Carefully open the packets to avoid any steam. Scatter fresh herbs over the shrimp before serving.

Kimi's Simple Grilled Fresh Fish

Servings: 2

Cooking Time: 45 Minutes

Ingredients:

- 1 Cup soy sauce
- 1/3 Cup extra-virgin olive oil
- 1 Tablespoon garlic, minced
- 2 lemons, juiced
- fresh basil
- 4 Pound Fresh Fish, cut into portion-sized pieces

Directions:

1. Mix all ingredients to create sauce and cover fish in marinade for 45 minutes.

2. Supply your smoker with wood pellets and follow the start-up procedure. Preheat the grill, with the lid closed, to 140° F. Grill the marinated fish on the grill until it reaches an internal temperature of 140-145°F. Serve immediately, enjoy! Grill: 350 °F Probe: 145 °F

Lemon Lobster Rolls

Servings: 4

Cooking Time: 35 Minutes

Ingredients:

- 1/2 Cup Butter
- 4 Hot Dog Bun(S)
- 1 Lemon, Whole
- 4 Lobster, Tail

➢ 1/4 Cup Mayo
➢ Pepper

Directions:

1. Supply your smoker with wood pellets and follow the start-up procedure. Preheat the grill, with the lid closed, to 300° F.

2. Using kitchen shears, cut the shell of the tail and crack in half so that the meat is exposed. Pour in butter and season with pepper. Place the tails meat side up on the grill and cook until the shell has turned red and the meat is white, about 35 minutes.

3. Remove from the grill and separate the shell from the meat. Place the meat in a bowl with mayo, lemon juice and rind and season with pepper. Stir to combine and evenly distribute into the hot dog buns.

Spicy Shrimp Skewers

Servings: 4
Cooking Time: 6 Minutes

Ingredients:

➢ 2 Pound shrimp, peeled and deveined
➢ 6 Thai chiles
➢ 6 Clove garlic
➢ 2 Tablespoon Winemaker's Napa Valley Rub
➢ 1 1/2 Teaspoon sugar
➢ 1 1/2 Tablespoon white vinegar
➢ 3 Tablespoon olive oil

Directions:

1. If using bamboo skewers, place them in cold water to soak for 1 hour before grilling.

2. Place shrimp in a bowl and set aside. Combine all remaining ingredients in a blender and blend until a coarse-textured paste is reached. Note: if a milder flavor is preferred, feel free to adjust amount of chiles to taste.

3. Add chile-garlic mixture to the shrimp and place in fridge to marinate for at least 30 minutes.

4. Remove from fridge and thread shrimp onto bamboo or metal skewers.

5. Supply your smoker with wood pellets and follow the start-up procedure. Preheat the grill, with the lid closed, to 450° F.

6. Place shrimp on grill and cook for 2 to 3 minutes per side or until shrimp are pink and firm to touch. Enjoy! Grill: 450 °F

Oysters In The Shell

Servings: 4
Cooking Time: 20 Minutes

Ingredients:

➢ 8 medium oysters, unopened, in the shell, rinsed and scrubbed
➢ 1 batch Lemon Butter Mop for Seafood

Directions:

1. Supply your smoker with wood pellets and follow the start-up procedure. Preheat the grill, with the lid closed, to 375°F.

2. Place the unopened oysters directly on the grill grate and grill for about 20 minutes, or until the oysters are done and their shells open.

3. Discard any oysters that do not open. Shuck the remaining oysters, transfer them to a bowl, and add the mop. Serve immediately.

Smoked Salt Cured Lox

Servings: 8
Cooking Time: 30 Minutes

Ingredients:

➢ 1 Cup kosher salt
➢ 1 Cup sugar
➢ 1 Tablespoon cracked black pepper
➢ 1 Whole lemon zest

- ➢ 1 Whole orange zest
- ➢ 1 Whole Packaged Dill, roughly chopped including stems
- ➢ 2 Pound salmon fillet, skin on

Directions:

1. Mix together salt, sugar, black pepper, lemon zest, orange zest, and dill.

2. Slice salmon in half. Coat all flesh of salmon completely with salt sugar mixture. Sandwich the 2 pieces together, flesh to flesh and completely cover with salt sugar mixture.

3. Wrap tightly with plastic wrap and place into a gallon zip top bag. Squeeze out as much air as possible. Place wrapped salmon into a baking dish and place something heavy on top like a pot filled with water or a brick wrapped in foil. Place into the refrigerator for 10 hours. After 10 hours, flip over and put the weight back on top. Refrigerate for another 10 hours.

4. Remove from refrigerator, unwrap and rinse of remaining salt with cold water. Pat dry and leave on counter for 1 hour.

5. Supply your smoker with wood pellets and follow the start-up procedure. Preheat the grill, with the lid closed, to 180° F.

6. Place salmon onto a baking pan. Fill another baking pan with ice and place baking pan with salmon over ice.

7. Place onto grill and smoke for 30 minutes. Remove from grill and slice thin. Grill: 180 ˚F

8. Serve with bagels, cream cheese, capers, dill, lemon wedges, sliced tomatoes, and red onion. Enjoy!

Sweet Mandarin Salmon

Servings: 2
Cooking Time: 10 Minutes

Ingredients:

- ➢ 1 Whole lime juice
- ➢ 1 Teaspoon sesame oil
- ➢ 1 1/2 Cup Mandarin Orange Sauce
- ➢ 1 1/2 Tablespoon soy sauce
- ➢ 2 Tablespoon cilantro, finely chopped
- ➢ Freshly cracked black pepper
- ➢ 1 Whole (4 oz) wild salmon fillets

Directions:

1. Supply your smoker with wood pellets and follow the start-up procedure. Preheat the grill, with the lid closed, to 375° F.

2. For the glaze, combine Mandarin orange sauce, lime juice, sesame oil, soy sauce, cilantro and fresh cracked black pepper. Mix together.

3. Cut the salmon into 4 fillets. Brush with glaze and place directly on the grill grate, skin side down.

4. Cook until salmon reaches an internal temperature of 155 degrees F (about 15-20 minutes). Half way through cook time, brush salmon again with the glaze.

5. Remove the salmon from the grill and serve with remaining glaze if desired. Enjoy!

Moules Marinières With Garlic Butter Sauce

Servings: 4
Cooking Time: 12 Minutes

Ingredients:

- ➢ 3lb (1.4kg) fresh mussels, scrubbed under cold running water and debearded
- ➢ lemon wedges
- ➢ crusty bread (optional)
- ➢ for the sauce
- ➢ 6 tbsp unsalted butter
- ➢ 3 garlic cloves, peeled and minced

- ➢ 1 cup dry white wine or hard cider
- ➢ 1 tbsp freshly squeezed lemon juice
- ➢ 2 tsp hot sauce, plus more
- ➢ coarse salt
- ➢ freshly ground black pepper
- ➢ 2 tbsp chopped fresh curly parsley or tarragon

Directions:

1. Supply your smoker with wood pellets and follow the start-up procedure. Preheat the grill, with the lid closed, to 450° F.

2. In a small saucepan on the stovetop over medium-low heat, make the sauce by melting the butter. Add the garlic and sauté for 1 to 2 minutes. Add the wine, lemon juice, and hot sauce. Season with salt and pepper to taste. Simmer for 5 minutes. Remove the saucepan from the heat and stir in the parsley. Keep warm.

3. Discard any mussels that are cracked or don't snap shut when tapped. Place the mussels in a large aluminum foil roasting pan and cover tightly with heavy-duty aluminum foil.

4. Place the pan on the grate and steam the mussels until the shells open, about 10 to 12 minutes. Remove the pan from the grill and use long-handled tongs to remove the foil from the pan. (Be careful of escaping steam.) Use the tongs to discard any mussels that don't open.

5. Pour the reserved garlic butter sauce over the mussels. Serve from the pan or transfer the mussels to a shallow serving bowl. Serve immediately with lemon wedges, additional hot sauce, and crusty bread (if using) to sop up the juices.

Dijon-smoked Halibut

Servings: 6
Cooking Time: 120 Minutes

Ingredients:

- ➢ 4 (6-ounce) halibut steaks
- ➢ ¼ cup extra-virgin olive oil
- ➢ 2 teaspoons kosher salt
- ➢ 1 teaspoon freshly ground black pepper
- ➢ ½ cup mayonnaise
- ➢ ½ cup sweet pickle relish
- ➢ ¼ cup finely chopped sweet onion
- ➢ ¼ cup chopped roasted red pepper
- ➢ ¼ cup finely chopped tomato
- ➢ ¼ cup finely chopped cucumber
- ➢ 2 tablespoons Dijon mustard
- ➢ 1 teaspoon minced garlic

Directions:

1. Rub the halibut steaks with the olive oil and season on both sides with the salt and pepper. Transfer to a plate, cover with plastic wrap, and refrigerate for 4 hours.

2. Supply your smoker with wood pellets and follow the start-up procedure. Preheat, with the lid closed, to 200°F.

3. Remove the halibut from the refrigerator and rub with the mayonnaise.

4. Put the fish directly on the grill grate, close the lid, and smoke for 2 hours, or until opaque and an instant-read thermometer inserted in the fish reads 140°F.

5. While the fish is smoking, combine the pickle relish, onion, roasted red pepper, tomato, cucumber, Dijon mustard, and garlic in a medium bowl. Refrigerate the mustard relish until ready to serve.

6. Serve the halibut steaks hot with the mustard relish.

Grilled Pepper Lobster Tails

Servings: 3
Cooking Time: 10 Minutes

Ingredients:

➢ Tt Black Pepper
➢ 3/4 Stick Butter, Room Temp
➢ 2 Tablespoons Chives, Chopped
➢ 1 Clove Garlic, Minced
➢ Lemon, Sliced
➢ 3 (7-Ounce) Lobster, Tail
➢ Tt Salt, Kosher

Directions:

1. Start your Grill on "SMOKE" with the lid open until a fire is established in the burn pot (3-7 minutes).
2. Supply your smoker with wood pellets and follow the start-up procedure. Preheat the grill, with the lid closed, to 350° F.
3. Blend butter, chives, minced garlic, and black pepper in a small bowl. Cover with plastic wrap and set aside.
4. Butterfly the tails down the middle of the softer underside of the shell. Don't cut entirely through the center of the meat. Brush the tails with olive oil and season with salt, to your liking.
5. Grill lobsters cut side down about 5 minutes until the shells are bright red in color. Flip the tails over and top with a generous tablespoon of herb butter. Grill for another 4 minutes, or until the lobster meat is an opaque white color.
6. Remove from the grill and serve with more herb butter and lemon wedges.

Cajun Catfish

Servings: 6
Cooking Time: 15 Minutes

Ingredients:

➢ 2½ pounds catfish fillets
➢ 2 tablespoons olive oil
➢ 1 batch Cajun Rub

Directions:

1. Supply your smoker with wood pellets and follow the start-up procedure. Preheat the grill, with the lid closed, to 300°F.
2. Coat the catfish fillets all over with olive oil and season with the rub. Using your hands, work the rub into the flesh.
3. Place the fillets directly on the grill grate and smoke until their internal temperature reaches 145°F. Remove the catfish from the grill and serve immediately

Smoked Cedar Plank Salmon

Servings: 4
Cooking Time: 20 Minutes

Ingredients:

➢ 1/4 Cup Brown Sugar
➢ 1/2 Tablespoon Olive Oil
➢ Competition Smoked Seasoning
➢ 4 Salmon Fillets, Skin Off

Directions:

1. Soak the untreated cedar plank in water for 24 hours before grilling. When ready to grill, remove and wipe down.
2. Supply your smoker with wood pellets and follow the start-up procedure. Preheat the grill, with the lid closed, to 350° F.
3. In a small bowl, mix the brown sugar, oil, and Lemon Pepper, Garlic, and Herb seasoning. Rub generously over the salmon fillets.
4. Place the plank over indirect heat, then lay the salmon on the plank and grill for 15-20 minutes, or until the salmon is cooked through and flakes easily with a fork. Remove from the heat and serve immediately.

Bbq Roasted Salmon

Servings: 4

Cooking Time: 15 Minutes

Ingredients:

- 1/3 Cup honey
- 3 Tablespoon Mustard, whole-grain
- 1 Cup ketchup
- 1/2 Cup dark brown sugar
- 1 Teaspoon Cider Vinegar
- 1/2 Teaspoon Thyme Leaves, finely chopped
- 1/8 Teaspoon Jacobsen Salt Co. Pure Kosher Sea Salt
- 1/8 Teaspoon freshly ground black pepper
- 4 Whole Salmon Fillets, 6oz each, skin-on

Directions:

1. Combine all sauce ingredients in a large bowl, preferably one day prior to making the salmon.
2. Rub salmon fillets on both sides with sauce. Reserve any extra, unused sauce.
3. Supply your smoker with wood pellets and follow the start-up procedure. Preheat the grill, with the lid closed, to 350° F.
4. Place fillets on grill, skin-side down, and cook for 15 minutes. Grill: 350 ˚F
5. Let the fish rest for about 3-5 minutes. Serve with extra sauce. Enjoy!

Traeger Jerk Shrimp

Servings: 8

Cooking Time: 10 Minutes

Ingredients:

- 1 Tablespoon brown sugar
- 1 Tablespoon smoked paprika
- 1 Teaspoon garlic powder
- 1/4 Teaspoon Thyme, ground
- 1/4 Teaspoon ground cayenne pepper
- 1 Teaspoon sea salt
- 1 lime zest
- 2 Pound shrimp in shell
- 3 Tablespoon olive oil

Directions:

1. Combine spices, salt, and lime zest in a small bowl and mix. Place shrimp into a large bowl, then drizzle in the olive oil, Add the spice mixture and toss to combine, making sure every shrimp is kissed with deliciousness.
2. Supply your smoker with wood pellets and follow the start-up procedure. Preheat the grill, with the lid closed, to 450° F.
3. Arrange the shrimp on the grill and cook for 2 – 3 minutes per side, until firm, opaque, and cooked through. Grill: 450 ˚F
4. Serve with lime wedges, fresh cilantro, mint, and Caribbean Hot Pepper Sauce. Enjoy!

Grilled Lobster Tails With Smoked Paprika Butter

Servings: 4

Cooking Time: 10-12 Minutes

Ingredients:

- 4 lobster tails, each about 8 to 10oz (225 to 285g), thawed if frozen
- 3 lemons, 1 quartered lengthwise, 2 halved through their equators
- for the butter
- 1¼ cup unsalted butter, at room temperature
- 2 garlic cloves, peeled and finely minced
- 3 tbsp chopped fresh parsley
- 2 tbsp chopped fresh chives
- 1 tbsp freshly squeezed lemon juice
- 2 tsp finely chopped lemon zest
- 2 tsp smoked paprika
- 1 tsp coarse salt

Directions:

1. Supply your smoker with wood pellets and follow the start-up procedure. Preheat the grill, with the lid closed, to 450° F.

2. In a medium bowl, make the paprika butter by combining the ingredients. Beat with a wooden spoon until well blended.

3. Use a sharp, heavy knife or sturdy kitchen shears to cut lengthwise through the top shell of each lobster tail in a straight line toward the tail fin. Gently loosen the meat from the bottom shell and sides. Lift the meat through the slit you just made so the meat sits on top of the shell. Slip a lemon quarter underneath the meat (between the meat and the bottom shell) to keep it elevated. Spread 1 tablespoon of paprika butter on top of each lobster. Melt the remaining butter and keep it warm.

4. Place the lobster tails flesh side up and lemon halves cut sides down on the grate. Grill the lobsters until the flesh is white and opaque and the internal temperature of the lobster meat reaches 135 to 140°F (57 to 60°C), about 10 to 12 minutes, basting at least once with some of the melted butter. (Don't overcook or the lobster will become unpleasantly rubbery.)

5. Transfer the lobsters and the lemon halves to a platter. Divide the remaining melted butter between 4 ramekins before serving.

Prosciutto-wrapped Scallops

Servings: 4
Cooking Time: 10 Minutes

Ingredients:

➢ 1½lb (680g) jumbo sea or diver scallops (size U-10)
➢ 8 to 10 thin slices of prosciutto, each halved lengthwise
➢ coarse salt
➢ freshly ground black pepper
➢ for the butter
➢ 8oz (225g) unsalted butter
➢ 2 tsp minced fresh curly or flat-leaf parsley
➢ 1½ tsp finely grated orange zest
➢ 1 tbsp freshly squeezed orange juice
➢ 1 tsp finely grated lemon zest
➢ 1 tsp finely grated lime zest
➢ ½ tsp coarse salt

Directions:

1. Supply your smoker with wood pellets and follow the start-up procedure. Preheat the grill, with the lid closed, to 450° F.

2. In a small saucepan on the stovetop over medium-low heat, make the citrus butter by melting the butter. Add the remaining ingredients and simmer for 3 to 5 minutes to blend the flavors. Keep warm.

3. Rinse the scallops under cold running water and dry with paper towels. Place each scallop on its side at the end of a piece of prosciutto and wrap the prosciutto around the scallop. Secure with a toothpick. Season the exposed sides of the scallop with salt and pepper.

4. Place the scallops exposed sides down on the grate and grill until the edges of the prosciutto begin to frizzle and the scallop is warm inside, about 3 to 5 minutes per side.

5. Transfer the scallops to a platter. Brush with some of the warm citrus butter before serving. Serve the remaining butter on the side.

Grilled Lemon Shrimp Scampi

Servings: 4
Cooking Time: 6 Minutes

Ingredients:

➢ 1½ pounds medium shrimp, peeled and deveined
➢ ¼ cup olive oil
➢ ¼ cup lemon juice
➢ 3 tablespoons chopped fresh parsley
➢ 1 tablespoon minced garlic
➢ ground black pepper to taste
➢ ¼ teaspoon crushed red pepper flakes to taste

Directions:

1. In a large, non-reactive bowl, stir together the olive oil, lemon juice, parsley, garlic, and black pepper. Season with crushed red pepper, if desired. Add shrimp, and toss to coat. Marinate in the refrigerator for 30 minutes.
2. Supply your smoker with wood pellets and follow the start-up procedure. Preheat the grill, with the lid closed, to high heat.
3. Thread shrimp onto skewers, piercing once near the tail and once near the head. Discard any remaining marinade.
4. Lightly oil grill grate. Place the shrimp skewers on the grill grates.
5. Grill for 2 to 3 minutes per side, or until opaque.

Whole Vermillion Red Snapper

Servings: 6
Cooking Time: 20 Minutes

Ingredients:

➢ 1 Whole Vermillion Red Snapper, scaled & gutted
➢ 4 Clove garlic, chopped
➢ 1 Whole lemon, thinly sliced
➢ 2 Sprig rosemary sprigs
➢ sea salt and freshly ground black pepper

Directions:

1. Supply your smoker with wood pellets and follow the start-up procedure. Preheat the grill, with the lid closed, to High heat.
2. Stuff the cavity of the fish with chopped garlic. Sprinkle the fish with sea salt, pepper, rosemary, and lemon.
3. Grill fish directly on the grill grate. Cook for 20-25 minutes. Serve. Enjoy!

Smoke-roasted Halibut With Mixed Herb Vinaigrette

Servings: 4
Cooking Time: 12 Minutes

Ingredients:

➢ 4 halibut fillets, each about 6 to 8oz (170 to 225g)
➢ for the vinaigrette
➢ 2 tbsp white wine vinegar or sherry vinegar, plus more
➢ ¼ tsp coarse salt, plus more
➢ ¼ tsp freshly ground black pepper, plus more
➢ ½ cup extra virgin olive oil
➢ 2 tbsp minced fresh herbs, such as dill, flat-leaf parsley, or oregano
➢ for serving
➢ 4 cups loosely packed baby arugula, spinach, or other mixed greens
➢ 1 lemon, cut lengthwise into 4 wedges

Directions:

1. Supply your smoker with wood pellets and follow the start-up procedure. Preheat the grill, with the lid closed, to 400° F.

2. In a small bowl, make the vinaigrette by whisking together the vinegar, and salt and pepper. Whisk until the salt dissolves. Continue to whisk while slowly adding the olive oil. Whisk until the vinaigrette is emulsified. Stir in the herbs. Taste, adding vinegar or salt and pepper to taste. Pour 1/3 of the vinaigrette into a separate container. Reserve the remainder.

3. Place the fillets on a rimmed sheet pan. Lightly brush both sides with the smaller portion of vinaigrette. (Dividing the vinaigrette into two containers prevents cross-contamination.) Lightly season with salt and pepper.

4. Place the fillets on the grate at an angle to the bars. Grill until the edges begin to look opaque, about 4 to 6 minutes. Gently turn and grill until the fish is cooked through, about 4 to 6 minutes more. (A fillet will break into clean flakes when pressed with a fork when it's done.)

5. Remove the fish from the grill. Place the greens in a large bowl and toss them with 2 to 3 tablespoons of the reserved vinaigrette (you want the greens lightly coated) and divide between 4 plates. Place a fillet on the greens on each plate. Drizzle a bit more of the vinaigrette over the top. Serve with lemon wedges.

Grilled Artichoke Cheese Salmon

Servings: 12

Cooking Time: 270 Minutes

Ingredients:
- 28 Oz Artichoke Hearts, Whole, Canned
- 1/2 Cup Breadcrumbs
- 1/2 Cup Brown Sugar
- 8 Oz Cream Cheese
- 1 Tbsp Garlic Powder
- 1 Cup Italian Cheese Blend, Shredded
- 1/4 Cup Kosher Salt
- 1 Cup Mayonnaise
- 2 Tsp Olive Oil
- 1 Tbsp Onion Powder
- 1/2 Cup Parmesan Cheese
- 2 Tbsp Parsley, Chopped
- Blackened Sriracha Rub
- 1 1/4 Lbs Salmon, Fillet, Scaled And Deboned
- Sour Cream
- 1/2 Tsp White Pepper, Ground

Directions:

1. In a small mixing bowl, whisk together the brown sugar, salt, garlic powder, onion powder, and white pepper. This will make twice the cure needed, so be sure and place the remaining half in a resealable plastic bag and save for smoking fish at a later date.

2. Lay a sheet of plastic wrap on a sheet tray and sprinkle a thin layer of the cure on it. Place the salmon skin-side down on top of the cure, then sprinkle a couple tablespoons of cure on top. Gently press the cure on top of the salmon flesh, then wrap in plastic wrap.

3. Refrigerate for 8 hours, or overnight.

4. Remove salmon from the refrigerator and wash off the cure in the sink, under cold water.

5. Blot salmon with a paper towel, then set salmon skin side on a wire rack. Dry at room temperature for two hours, or until a yellowish shimmer appears on the salmon.

6. Supply your smoker with wood pellets and follow the start-up procedure. Preheat the grill, with the lid closed, to 250° F. If using a gas, charcoal or other grill, set it to low, indirect heat.

7. Place the salmon in the upper cabinet. Smoke for 2 hours, then increase the grill temperature to

350° F to maintain a cabinet temperature of 225°F and smoke another 1 to 2 hours, until salmon reaches an internal temperature of 145° F.

8. Remove salmon from the cabinet and set aside to rest for 15 minutes, then flake apart. Reserve ½ cup to top dip after grilling.

9. While the salmon is resting, drain the artichokes, then skewer onto metal skewers (if using wooden skewers, make sure to soak in water for 1 hour prior to grilling, or you can use a grill basket as well).

10. Season with Blackened Sriracha, then set on the grill. Grill for 2 to 3 minutes, until lightly browned.

11. Remove from the grill, cool slightly, then roughly chop. Set aside.

12. In a mixing bowl, combine shredded Italian cheese, grated parmesan, breadcrumbs and parsley. Set aside.

13. Place cream cheese, mayonnaise, and sour cream in a cast iron skillet. Stir frequently, with a wooden spoon, for about 5 minutes, until the mixture is smooth.

14. Carefully fold in flaked salmon and grilled artichoke hearts, then spread breadcrumb mixture over dip.

15. Drizzle with olive oil, then close the grill lid and bake for 25 to 30 minutes, until dip begins to bubble around the edges, and cheese begins to caramelize on top.

16. Remove dip from the grill, top with reserved salmon and a pinch of parsley. Serve warm with bagel chips, crackers, or crusty bread.

Grilled Trout With Citrus & Basil

Servings: 4

Cooking Time: 10 Minutes

Ingredients:

- 6 Whole Trout
- 2 Teaspoon Blackened Saskatchewan Rub
- 10 Sprig fresh basil
- 2 Lemons, cut in half
- extra-virgin olive oil

Directions:

1. Supply your smoker with wood pellets and follow the start-up procedure. Preheat the grill, with the lid closed, to 450° F.

2. Season the center cavity of the trout with the Traeger Blackened Saskatchewan. Place two sprigs of Basil in each cavity, then add 4 lemon halves.

3. Next tie the fish closed using the Butchers twine, and then rub with olive oil.

4. Place the trout on the hot grill and cook 5 minutes on each side. Enjoy! Grill: 450 ˚F

Smoked Lobster Scampi

Servings: 2

Cooking Time: 30 Minutes

Ingredients:

- 1 Lobster Tail
- 1 Handful Pasta, Angel Hair
- 2 Tablespoon butter
- 1 Teaspoon garlic, minced
- 1/2 Teaspoon lemon juice
- 2 Teaspoon Parmesan cheese, grated
- 2 Tablespoon Sun Dried Tomato Pesto
- fresh parsley

Directions:

1. Supply your smoker with wood pellets and follow the start-up procedure. Preheat the grill, with the lid closed, to 180° F.

2. Use kitchen shears to cut along the top of the lobster on both sides to expose the meat. Place the lobster directly on the grill for 20-25 minutes, depending on the size of the lobster. Grill: 180 ˚F

3. While lobster smokes, cook pasta according to packaged directions.

4. After 20-25 minutes, take lobster off the grill and remove the meat from the tail. Cut meat into chunks.

5. While the pasta is boiling, melt butter over medium high heat. Once butter starts to brown, add the garlic and lobster chunks. Toss in pan a few times then add lemon and parmesan. Set aside.

6. When pasta has finished, place 1 tbsp of the sun dried tomato pesto on the bottom of a bowl or plate. Top with pasta, then finish with the lobster scampi. Garnish with parsley. Enjoy!

PORK RECIPES

Honey Glazed Pork Chops

Servings: 6
Cooking Time: 16 Minutes

Ingredients:
- 4-6 Pork Chop
- 1/2 Cup of Honey
- 4 Tablespoons Soy Sauce
- 2 Tablespoons Olive Oil
- 2 Garlic Cloves, pressed
- Salt & Pepper

Directions:
1. Supply your smoker with wood pellets and follow the start-up procedure. Preheat the grill, with the lid closed, to 350° F.
2. Mix together the honey, soy sauce, and garlic in a small dish.
3. Brush the olive oil over the pork chops and sprinkle with salt and pepper.
4. Place the pork chops on the grill and brush the honey mixture over the top side.
5. When you flip the pork chops over, brush the second side with the honey mixture.
6. Grill for about 8 minutes on each side or until a thermometer inserted reads 170 degrees. Brush a final layer of the honey glaze over the pork chops before serving. Enjoy!

Traeger Smoked Sausage

Servings: 4
Cooking Time: 120 Minutes

Ingredients:
- 3 Pound ground pork
- 1/2 Tablespoon ground mustard
- 1 Tablespoon onion powder
- 1 Tablespoon garlic powder
- 1/2 Teaspoon pink curing salt
- 1 Tablespoon salt
- 4 Teaspoon black pepper
- 1/2 Cup ice water
- Hog casings, soaked and rinsed in cold water

Directions:
1. In a medium bowl, combine the meat and seasonings, mix well.
2. Add ice water to meat and mix with hands working quickly until everything is incorporated.
3. Place mixture in a sausage stuffer and follow manufacturers Directions:for operating. Use caution not to overstuff or the casing might burst.
4. Once all the meat is stuffed, determine your desired link length and pinch and twist a couple of times or tie it off. Repeat for each link.
5. Supply your smoker with wood pellets and follow the start-up procedure. Preheat the grill, with the lid closed, to 225° F.
6. Place links directly on the grill grate and cook for 1 to 2 hours or until the internal temperature registers 155°F. Let sausage rest a few minutes before slicing. Enjoy! Grill: 225 °F Probe: 155 °F

Bbq Pork Shoulder Roast With Sugar Lips Glaze

Servings: 8
Cooking Time: 540 Minutes

Ingredients:
- 1 (8-10 lb) bone-in pork butt
- 1/4 Cup Pork & Poultry Rub, divided
- 1 1/2 Cup apple juice, divided

- ➢ 4 Tablespoon brown sugar
- ➢ 1 Tablespoon salt
- ➢ 1/2 Cup apple juice
- ➢ Sugar Lips Glaze

Directions:

1. Trim pork butt of all excess fat leaving 1/4 inch of the fat cap attached.

2. Combine 2 tablespoons Traeger Pork & Poultry Rub, 1 cup apple juice, brown sugar and salt in a small bowl stirring until most of the sugar and salt are dissolved. Inject the pork butt every square inch or so with the apple juice mixture.

3. Season the exterior of the pork butt with remaining Traeger Pork & Poultry Rub.

4. Supply your smoker with wood pellets and follow the start-up procedure. Preheat the grill, with the lid closed, to 250° F.

5. Place pork butt directly on the grill grate and cook for about 6 hours or until the internal temperature reaches 160°F. Grill: 250 °F Probe: 160 °F

6. Wrap the pork butt in two layers of foil and pour in 1/2 cup of apple juice. Secure tin foil tightly to contain the apple juice.

7. Increase Traeger temperature to 275°F and return wrapped pork butt to grill in a pan large enough to hold the pork butt in case it leaks. Cook an additional 3 hours or until internal temperature reaches 195°F. Grill: 275 °F Probe: 195 °F

8. Remove from the grill and allow to rest 10 to 15 minutes. Slice the pork butt around the bone and top with Traeger Sugar Lips BBQ Sauce. Serve with your favorite sides. Enjoy!

Grilled Bratwurst With Apple Slaw

Servings: 2
Cooking Time: 20 Minutes

Ingredients:

- ➢ 2 Whole Granny Smith Apples, Unpeeled
- ➢ 1/2 Small Red Onion, peeled
- ➢ 1/2 Cup mayonnaise
- ➢ 1/2 Tablespoon apple cider vinegar
- ➢ 1/4 Cup spicy brown mustard
- ➢ 1 Teaspoon Veggie Rub
- ➢ 1 Stick butter, melted
- ➢ 6 Whole bratwurst
- ➢ 6 Whole buns

Directions:

1. Supply your smoker with wood pellets and follow the start-up procedure. Preheat the grill, with the lid closed, to 350° F. For the apple slaw: Grate unpeeled Granny Smith apples and red onion into a large bowl. Toss with mayonnaise, apple cider vinegar, spicy brown mustard, Traeger Veggie Rub and melted butter.

2. Place brats directly on the grill grate and cook for 10 minutes per side, or when an instant read thermometer inserted into the thickest part of the meat registers 160 degrees F. Grill: 350 °F Probe: 160 °F

3. Remove from grill, place in bun and top with apple slaw. Enjoy!

Smoked Spare Ribs

Servings: 4-8
Cooking Time: 360 Minutes

Ingredients:

- ➢ 2 (2- or 3-pound) racks spare ribs
- ➢ 2 tablespoons yellow mustard

- ➢ 1 batch Sweet Brown Sugar Rub
- ➢ ¼ cup The Ultimate BBQ Sauce

Directions:

1. Supply your smoker with wood pellets and follow the start-up procedure. Preheat the grill, with the lid closed, to 225°F.

2. Remove the membrane from the backside of the ribs. This can be done by cutting just through the membrane in an X pattern and working a paper towel between the membrane and the ribs to pull it off.

3. Coat the ribs on both sides with mustard and season with the rub. Using your hands, work the rub into the meat.

4. Place the ribs directly on the grill grate and smoke until their internal temperature reaches between 190°F and 200°F.

5. Baste both sides of the ribs with barbecue sauce.

6. Increase the grill's temperature to 300°F and continue to cook the ribs for 15 minutes more.

7. Remove the racks from the grill, cut them into individual ribs, and serve immediately.

Hawaiian Pulled Pig

Servings: 4

Cooking Time: 300 Minutes

Ingredients:

- ➢ 7 Pound bone-in pork shoulder
- ➢ 3 Tablespoon Jacobsen Salt Co. Pure Kosher Sea Salt
- ➢ ground black pepper
- ➢ 2 Whole Banana Leaves

Directions:

1. Season the pork shoulder with Jacobsen Salt and pepper.

2. Place a banana leaf on your work surface. Lay the pork shoulder in the center of it, and draw up the ends as if you were wrapping a gift. Lay the second banana leaf at right angles to the first and draw up the ends to enclose the meat. Wrap the entire package tightly in aluminum foil. Refrigerate overnight.

3. Supply your smoker with wood pellets and follow the start-up procedure. Preheat the grill, with the lid closed, to 300° F.

4. Place the wrapped pork directly on the grill grate and cook until the pork is falling-apart-tender, 5 to 6 hours, or until it has reached an internal temperature of 190 degrees F. Grill: 300 °F Probe: 190 °F

5. Transfer the pork to a cutting board and let rest, still wrapped, for 20 minutes. Carefully unwrap the pork and save any juices that accumulated in the foil.

6. Tear the pork into chunks and shreds, discarding any lumps of fat or bone. Enjoy!

Jamaican Jerk Pork Chops

Servings: 4

Cooking Time: 720 Minutes

Ingredients:

- ➢ 4 thick pork rib or loin chops, each about 12oz (340g) and 1 inch (2.5cm) thick
- ➢ for the marinade
- ➢ ½ to 1 Scotch bonnet or habanero pepper, destemmed, deseeded, and coarsely chopped, plus more
- ➢ 2 scallions, trimmed, white and green parts coarsely chopped
- ➢ 1 garlic clove, peeled and coarsely chopped
- ➢ juice of 1 lime
- ➢ 2 tbsp vegetable oil

- ➢ 2 tbsp distilled water
- ➢ 1 tbsp light soy sauce
- ➢ 2 tsp coarsely chopped fresh thyme leaves
- ➢ 2 tsp peeled and minced fresh ginger
- ➢ 2 tsp dark brown sugar or low-carb substitute, plus more
- ➢ 1 tsp coarse salt, plus more
- ➢ ½ tsp freshly ground black pepper
- ➢ ½ tsp ground allspice
- ➢ ½ tsp ground nutmeg
- ➢ ½ tsp ground cinnamon

Directions:

1. In a blender, make the jerk marinade by combining the ingredients. Blend until fairly smooth. Taste for seasoning, adding more Scotch bonnet, brown sugar, or salt. Place the pork chops in a resealable plastic bag and pour the marinade over them, turning and massaging the bag to thoroughly coat the meat. Refrigerate for 2 to 4 hours.

2. Supply your smoker with wood pellets and follow the start-up procedure. Preheat the grill, with the lid closed, to 425° F.

3. Remove the pork from the marinade and scrape off the excess. (Discard the marinade.) Grill the chops until the internal temperature reaches 145°F (63°C), about 6 to 8 minutes per side.

4. Transfer the chops to a platter. Let rest for 2 minutes before serving.

Bbq Pork Shoulder Steaks

Servings: 4
Cooking Time: 120 Minutes

Ingredients:

- ➢ 4 (1 to 1-1/4 inch thick) pork shoulder steaks
- ➢ 1/2 Cup mustard
- ➢ Pork & Poultry Rub
- ➢ 1/2 Cup apple juice
- ➢ 1 Cup 'Que BBQ Sauce

Directions:

1. Slather the pork steaks on all sides with the mustard and season with the Traeger Pork & Poultry Rub. (The mustard will help keep the pork moist, but the taste will be unnoticeable in the final product.)

2. Supply your smoker with wood pellets and follow the start-up procedure. Preheat the grill, with the lid closed, to 180° F.

3. Arrange the steaks on the grill grate. Smoke for 1-1/2 hours. Grill: 180 ˚F

4. Remove the pork steaks to a plate and increase temperature to 225°F. Preheat 5 to 10 minutes. Grill: 225 ˚F

5. Meanwhile, wrap each steak with aluminum foil, adding in a couple tablespoons of apple juice.

6. Cook the steaks for another hour or so or until they are tender (about 160°F on an instant-read meat thermometer). Grill: 225 ˚F Probe: 160 ˚F

7. The last 15 minutes, take the pork steaks out of the foil and put them directly on the grill.

8. Brush each steak on both sides with the Traeger 'Que BBQ Sauce or your favorite barbecue sauce.

9. Let the steaks rest for 3 minutes before serving. Enjoy!

Smoked Curry Ketchup Pork Ribs

Servings: 4
Cooking Time: 205 Minutes

Ingredients:

- ➢ 1 Tsp Chili Powder
- ➢ 1 Tbsp Curry Powder

- ➢ 1/2 Tsp Ground Mustard
- ➢ 2 Tsp Honey
- ➢ To Taste, Kansas City Barbecue Rub Seasoning
- ➢ 1 Cup Ketchup
- ➢ 2 Pork Back Rib Racks, Membrane Removed
- ➢ 2 Tsp Smoked Paprika
- ➢ 2 Tsp Worcestershire Sauce

Directions:

1. Supply your smoker with wood pellets and follow the start-up procedure. Preheat the grill, with the lid open, to 225° F. If using a gas or charcoal grill, set it up for low, indirect heat.
2. Place rib racks on a sheet tray, then season both sides with Kansas City Barbeque Rub. Transfer ribs to the grill and smoke for 1 hour.
3. Meanwhile, prepare the curry ketchup: In a mixing bowl, add ketchup, curry powder, smoked paprika, chili powder, ground mustard, Worcestershire, and honey and whisk to incorporate. Set aside.
4. Rotate the rib racks and increase temperature to 250 F. Cook for another hour, then remove the ribs from the grill and place on butcher paper. Brush ribs with sauce then wrap with paper.
5. Return ribs to the grill. Cook for one more hour, until tender.
6. Remove ribs from the grill, cut open the butcher paper, and baste with remaining curry ketchup. Place racks back on the grill, increase the temperature to 275 F, then cook for an additional 15 minutes. Remove ribs from the grill, cut open the butcher paper, and baste with remaining curry ketchup. Place racks back on the grill, increase the temperature to 275 F, then cook for an additional 15 minutes.
7. Remove ribs from the grill, rest for 10 minutes, then slice and serve warm.

Maple-smoked Pork Chops

Servings: 4
Cooking Time: 55 Minutes

Ingredients:

- ➢ 1 (12-pound) full packer brisket
- ➢ 2 tablespoons yellow mustard
- ➢ 1 batch Espresso Brisket Rub
- ➢ Worcestershire Mop and Spritz, for spritzing

Directions:

1. Supply your smoker with wood pellets and follow the start-up procedure. Preheat the grill, with the lid closed, to 180°F.
2. Season the pork chops on both sides with salt and pepper.
3. Place the chops directly on the grill grate and smoke for 30 minutes.
4. Increase the grill's temperature to 350°F. Continue to cook the chops until their internal temperature reaches 145°F.
5. Remove the pork chops from the grill and let them rest for 5 minutes before serving.

Bbq Pulled Pork With Sweet & Heat Bbq Sauce

Servings: 4
Cooking Time: 540 Minutes

Ingredients:

- ➢ 10 Pound Bone-In Pork Butt
- ➢ 2 Tablespoon Pork & Poultry Rub
- ➢ 1 1/2 Cup apple juice
- ➢ 4 Tablespoon brown sugar
- ➢ 1 Tablespoon salt
- ➢ 1 To Taste salt

- ➢ 1 To Taste Pork & Poultry Rub
- ➢ 1 As Needed Sweet & Heat BBQ Sauce

Directions:

1. Trim pork butt of all excess fat leaving 1/4" of the fat cap attached. Combine 2 Tbsp Pork and Poultry rub, apple juice, brown sugar, and salt in a small bowl stirring until most of the sugar and salt are dissolved. Inject the pork butt every square inch or so with the apple juice mixture. Season the exterior of the pork butt with remaining rub.

2. Supply your smoker with wood pellets and follow the start-up procedure. Preheat the grill, with the lid closed, to 225° F.

3. Place pork butt directly on the grill grate and cook for about 6 hours or until the internal temperature reaches 160°F. Grill: 225 °F Probe: 160 °F

4. Wrap the pork butt in two layers of foil and pour in 1/2 cup of apple juice. Secure tin foil tightly to contain the apple juice. Increase temperature to 275°F and return to grill in a pan large enough to hold the pork butt in case of leaks. Cook an additional 3 hours or until internal temperature reaches 205°F. Grill: 275 °F Probe: 205 °F

5. Remove from the grill and discard the bone. Shred the pork removing any excess fat or tendons. Season with additional Pork and Poultry Rub and salt if needed.

6. Add Sweet & Heat BBQ sauce and serve. Enjoy!

Grilled Stuffed Pork Chops

Servings: 4
Cooking Time: 45 Minutes

Ingredients:

- ➢ 4 Whole Pork, Loins
- ➢ 2 Cup Herb-Seasoned or Cornbread Stuffing Mix
- ➢ Apples, chopped
- ➢ onion, chopped
- ➢ Celery, Chopped
- ➢ chopped sage
- ➢ Pork & Poultry Rub or salt and pepper

Directions:

1. Cut a deep pocket in the side of each chop with a small sharp knife, cutting toward the bone but not all the way through.

2. Prepare the stuffing mix according to the package directions, adding your own touches if desired (try adding in chopped onion, a stalk of chopped celery, a finely diced apple, a few leaves of chopped sage and about 4 oz browned sausage).

3. Generously stuff each pork chop pocket with the mixture. Season both sides of the chops with Traeger Pork and Poultry Rub.

4. Supply your smoker with wood pellets and follow the start-up procedure. Preheat the grill, with the lid closed, to 325° F.

5. Arrange the chops directly on the grill grate. Bake for 45 to 50 minutes, or until the chops reach an internal temperature of 160 degrees F. There is no need to turn the chops.

6. Let the pork rest for 2 to 3 minutes before transferring to a platter or plates. Enjoy!

Roasted Ham With Apricot Sauce

Servings: 8
Cooking Time: 120 Minutes

Ingredients:

- ➢ 1 (8-10 lb) Snake River Farms Kurobuta Whole Bone-In Ham
- ➢ 1 Bottle Apricot BBQ Sauce

- ➢ 1/4 Cup horseradish
- ➢ 2 Tablespoon Dijon mustard

Directions:

1. Supply your smoker with wood pellets and follow the start-up procedure. Preheat the grill, with the lid closed, to 325° F.

2. Place ham in a large roasting pan lined with aluminum foil. Place pan on grill and cook for 90 minutes. Grill: 325 °F

3. For the Glaze: In a saucepan over medium heat, combine the Traeger Apricot BBQ Sauce, horseradish and mustard. Set aside and keep warm.

4. After 90 minutes, brush the ham with the glaze. Continue to cook for another 30 minutes or until a thermometer inserted into the thickest part of the ham reaches an internal temperatures of 135°F. Grill: 325 °F Probe: 135 °F

5. Remove ham from grill and rest for 20 minutes before slicing.

6. Serve with remaining glaze if desired. Enjoy!

Baby Back Ribs

Servings: 12-15
Cooking Time: 360 Minutes

Ingredients:

- ➢ 2 full slabs baby back ribs, back membranes removed
- ➢ 1 cup prepared table mustard
- ➢ 1 cup Pork Rub
- ➢ 1 cup apple juice, divided
- ➢ 1 cup packed light brown sugar, divided
- ➢ 1 cup of The Ultimate BBQ Sauce, divided

Directions:

1. Supply your smoker with wood pellets and follow the start-up procedure. Preheat, with the lid closed, to 150° to 180°F, or to the "Smoke" setting.

2. Coat the ribs with the mustard to help the rub stick and lock in moisture.

3. Generously apply the rub

4. Place the ribs directly on the grill, close the lid, and smoke for 3 hours5. Increase the temperature to 225°F.

5. Remove the ribs from the grill and wrap each rack individually with aluminum foil, but before sealing tightly, add ½ cup apple juice and ½ cup brown sugar to each package

6. Return the foil-wrapped ribs to the grill, close the lid, and smoke for 2 more hours.

7. Carefully unwrap the ribs and remove the foil completely. Coat each slab with ½ cup of barbecue sauce and continue smoking with the lid closed for 30 minutes to 1 hour, or until the meat tightens and has a reddish bark. For the perfect rack, the internal temperature should be 190°F.

Grilled Bbq Pork Chops

Servings: 6
Cooking Time: 12 Minutes

Ingredients:

- ➢ 6 Thick-Cut Pork Chops
- ➢ Generous amounts BBQ rub

Directions:

1. Supply your smoker with wood pellets and follow the start-up procedure. Preheat the grill, with the lid closed, to 450° F. Place seasoned pork chops on grill. Cook 6 minutes per side, or until internal temps reach 145 °F.

2. Remove from heat and let sit for 5-10 minutes before serving.

Smoked Ribs

Servings: 4
Cooking Time: 315 Minutes

Ingredients:

➢ 2 Racks Baby Back Rib
➢ Sweet Rib Rub

Directions:

1. Supply your smoker with wood pellets and follow the start-up procedure. Preheat the grill, with the lid open, to 225° F.

2. Remove the membrane on the reverse side of the ribs by sliding a butter knife under the membrane and breaking it. With a piece of paper towel, grab the broken membrane and peel back until the entire membrane is removed.

3. Season both sides of the ribs with Sweet Rib Rub.

4. Place the ribs, meat side up, on the grates of the grill and close the lid. Smoke for about 4 1/2 hours.

5. Wrap in foil and return to the grill at 350°F for another 45 minutes.

6. Pull your ribs off the grill and rest for 10 minutes.

7. Slice and serve hot. Enjoy!

Grilled Lasagna With Cold-smoked Mozzarella

Servings: 8-12
Cooking Time: 70 Minutes

Ingredients:

➢ 15 Oz. Ricotta Cheese
➢ 3 Cups Cold-Smoked Mozzarella, Grated Divided
➢ 2 Eggs
➢ 6 Garlic Cloves, Chopped
➢ 1 Tsp Garlic Powder
➢ 1 Cup Grated Parmesan Cheese, Divided
➢ 1 Lb. Italian Sausage
➢ 1 Tbsp Italian Seasoning
➢ 1 Pkg. "No-Bake" Lasagna Noodles
➢ 48 Oz. Marinara Sauce
➢ 1 Lb. Mozzarella Block
➢ 1 Tbsp Olive Oil
➢ 1 Tbsp Chopped Oregano
➢ ¼ Cup Italian Parsley, Chopped
➢ 1 Yellow Onion, Chopped

Directions:

1. In a glass bowl, mix together the eggs, Italian seasoning, garlic powder, ricotta cheese, ½ cup parmesan cheese, and 1 cup of smoked mozzarella, and 2 tablespoons of parsley. Cover and refrigerate for 1 hour.

2. Supply your smoker with wood pellets and follow the start-up procedure. Preheat the grill, with the lid open, to 400° F. If using a gas or charcoal grill, set it up for medium-high heat. Place a cast iron skillet on the grill grates and allow to preheat.

3. Heat olive oil in skillet, then add Italian sausage and cook for 5 minutes, then add in onion and garlic, and cook an additional 3 minutes. Remove from heat and stir in 1 tablespoon of parsley and dried oregano. Set aside and reduce grill temperature to 350° F.

4. To assemble, begin by covering the bottom of a 9x13 pan with 1 cup of sauce. For the first layer, place a single layer of uncooked noodles over the sauce, followed by ⅓ of the ricotta cheese mixture, half of the Italian sausage, 1 cup of mozzarella cheese, and 1 cup of sauce. Repeat for layer two with a single layer of uncooked lasagna noodles, ⅓ of the ricotta cheese mixture, and 1 ½ cups of

sauce. Repeat for layer three with a layer of uncooked lasagna noodles, remaining ricotta mixture, remaining Italian sausage, 1 cup of sauce. For the final layer, add a layer of uncooked lasagna noodles, remaining sauce, and remaining 1 cup mozzarella plus ½ cup parmesan.

5. Transfer lasagna to grill and cook, covered with foil, for 35 minutes. Remove foil and continue cooking for 10 minutes, sprinkle with additional parmesan and parsley, if desired. Remove from grill and let stand 15 minutes before serving.

Double-decker Pulled Pork Nachos With Smoked Cheese

Servings: 4
Cooking Time: 55 Minutes

Ingredients:
- 8 Ounce pepper jack cheese
- 8 Ounce Cheese, sharp cheddar
- tortilla chips
- 2 Cup leftover pulled pork
- black olives
- jalapeño, diced
- cilantro

Directions:
1. Supply your smoker with wood pellets and follow the start-up procedure. Preheat the grill, with the lid closed, to 165° F.
2. Place the cheese (frozen) on a rack on top of a tray filled with ice. You may want to cut the cheese into smaller portions, maybe 2 or 3 chunks per block, to help it smoke more quickly.
3. Smoke the cheeses for 45 to 60 minutes; allow to cool. Shred the cheeses (about 1 cup of each), and set aside. Grill: 165 ˚F

4. Turn the heat on the Traeger up to 350 degrees and preheat, lid closed, for 10 to 15 minutes. Grill: 350 ˚F
5. Lay out your tortilla chips on large baking sheet and top evenly with the shredded, smoked cheeses. Place the baking sheet on the Traeger grill grate and cook for about 10 minutes, or until the cheese is melted and bubbly. Grill: 350 ˚F
6. Remove the pan from the Traeger and start to assemble the double-decker nachos. Assemble the nachos with a layer of cheesy chips on the bottom, some pulled pork, and more cheesy chips on top. Finish it off with your favorite nacho toppings. Serve warm.

Pork & Pepperoni Burgers

Servings: 4
Cooking Time: 60 Minutes

Ingredients:
- 1lb (450g) bulk pork sausage, preferably Italian
- 1lb (450g) ground pork, well chilled
- 8 slices of bacon, preferably thick-cut
- 8oz (225g) grated mozzarella cheese, plus more
- 1 tsp Italian seasoning
- ½ cup pizza sauce
- 1½oz (40g) pepperoni, roughly chopped

Directions:
1. Wet your hands with cold water. In a large bowl, combine the sausage and ground pork until well mixed. Line a rimmed sheet pan with aluminum foil. Divide the meat into 4 equal-sized balls and place on the sheet pan. Spray the lower third of a soda can (including the bottom) with cooking spray. Firmly press the can into one of the meatballs to create a meat bowl with uniform

sides. Gently twist or rock the can to remove. Use your hands to repair any cracks in the bowl.

2. Wrap 2 slices of bacon around the circumference of the bowl and secure with toothpicks. Repeat with the remaining meatballs, respraying the can with cooking spray as necessary. Chill for 1 hour.

3. Supply your smoker with wood pellets and follow the start-up procedure. Preheat the grill, with the lid closed, to 300° F.

4. Place the patties cup side up on the grate and grill for 30 minutes. Use paper towels to blot any grease that pools at the bottom of the cups.

5. Sprinkle 2 tablespoons of cheese into each cup. Top each patty with equal amounts of Italian seasoning, pizza sauce, and pepperoni. Generously sprinkle more cheese over the top. Continue to grill until the bacon crisps, the cheese melts, and the internal temperature reaches 160°F (71°C), about 20 to 30 minutes more.

6. Remove the burgers from the grill and rest for 3 minutes. Remove the toothpicks and serve immediately.

Smoked Apple Pork Belly

Servings: 12
Cooking Time: 370 Minutes

Ingredients:
- 4 Pounds Slab Pork Belly (Uncured)
- 2 Cups Apple Juice (Divided Use)
- ½ Cup BBQ Sauce
- ¼ Cup Signature Sweet Rub

Directions:
1. Supply your smoker with wood pellets and follow the start-up procedure. Preheat the grill, with the lid closed, to 250° F.

2. Score the top layer of fat on the pork belly in 1 inch squares. Don't cut too deep, just barely into the muscle. Season liberally with the Sweet Rub on all sides.

3. Place the seasoned pork belly on the grill and smoke until the internal temperature reaches 165 degrees F (about 6 hours). Spritz with the apple juice every hour while it is cooking.

4. Once the belly reaches 165 degrees F, remove from the grill and wrap in heavy duty tinfoil with 1/2 cup of the apple juice. Seal the edges of the foil completely and return to the grill until the internal temperature reaches 200 degrees F.

5. Carefully remove the belly from the foil and drizzle with the apple juices from the foil. Return the pork belly to the grill and brush with BBQ sauce. Cook on the grill for 10 more minutes.

6. Remove the finished pork belly from the grill and let it rest for 10-15 more minutes before serving.

Amazing Bacon Cheese Fries

Servings: 2
Cooking Time: 25 Minutes

Ingredients:
- 2 Bacon, Strip
- 1/2 Cup Colby Jack Cheese, Shredded
- 1/2 Package Fries, Frozen
- 1/2 Cup Monterey Jack Cheese, Shredded

Directions:
1. Supply your smoker with wood pellets and follow the start-up procedure. Preheat the grill, with the lid open, to 350° F.

2. Place the bacon on the bacon rack and place on the grill. Cook until crispy, about 15 minutes.

3. Once slightly cooled, crumble the strips into small pieces and set it aside.

4. Grill the frozen French fries based on the package instructions, cooking on a pan in the instead of the oven.

5. Once fries are golden brown, sprinkle cheese and bacon on top of the fries, and return the pan to the grill and barbecue at 450°F for 1 minute. Remove from grill and enjoy!

Spiced Coffee-rubbed Ribs

Servings: 6 - 8

Cooking Time: 360 Minutes

Ingredients:

- 1 Tbsp Ancho Chili Powder
- Ground Black Pepper
- ½ Tsp Cocoa Powder
- 2 Tbsp Coffee
- ½ Tsp Coriander, Ground
- 1 Tbsp Dark Brown Sugar
- 1 Tsp Garlic Powder
- 2 Tbsp Kosher Salt
- 1 Tsp Onion Powder
- 1 Tsp Oregano
- 2 Tbsp Paprika
- 8 Lbs. Pork Spareribs

Directions:

1. Begin by preparing the dry rub. In a mixing bowl, whisk together the coffee, salt, paprika, brown sugar, oregano, garlic powder, onion powder, black pepper, cocoa powder and coriander. Set aside.

2. Remove the membrane from the back of your ribs: Take a butter knife and wedge it just underneath the membrane to loosen it. Using your hands or a paper towel to grip, pull the membrane up and off the bone. Place the ribs on a sheet tray, then rub each rack generously with dry rub. Wrap ribs in foil, then refrigerate overnight.

3. When ready to cook, remove ribs from the refrigerator and let come to room temp. Supply your smoker with wood pellets and follow the start-up procedure. Preheat the grill, with the lid open, to 225° F. If using a gas or charcoal grill, set it up for low indirect heat.

4. Place foil-wrapped ribs on the grill and close lid. Cook for 4 hours then remove foil from ribs and pour accumulated juices into a glass measuring cup. Pour the sauce over the ribs, then continue to cook for an additional 1 ½ - 2 hours or until tender. Remove from grill, slice and serve.

Grilled German Sausage With A Smoky Traeger Twist

Servings: 8

Cooking Time: 120 Minutes

Ingredients:

- 2 Tablespoon Jacobsen Salt Co. Pure Kosher Sea Salt
- 1 Teaspoon The Sausage Maker Instacure #1
- 1 Tablespoon ground nutmeg
- 2 Teaspoon ground mace
- 1 Teaspoon ground ginger
- 4 Pound ground pork, 80% lean
- 1 Pound ground veal or ground beef
- 2 Large eggs
- 1 Cup nonfat dry milk powder

Directions:

1. Combine salt, Instacure #1, nutmeg, mace and ginger in a large pitcher or small bowl. Add the milk and eggs. Beat until well combined. Pour the egg mixture over the ground meat and mix gently. Using your hands, mix in the milk powder until evenly distributed.

2.   Form the meat into sausage links, roughly 4 to 6 inches in length.

3.   Supply your smoker with wood pellets and follow the start-up procedure. Preheat the grill, with the lid closed, to 225° F.

4.   Smoke for approximately 2 hours, or until the internal temperature reaches 175°F. Serve immediately or refrigerate until ready to serve. Enjoy! Grill: 225 °F Probe: 175 °F

Bbq Baby Back Ribs With Bacon Pineapple Glaze By Scott Thomas

Servings: 4

Cooking Time: 180 Minutes

Ingredients:

- 2 Rack baby back ribs
- 1 As Needed salt and pepper
- 1 As Needed Your Favorite Spicy Rub
- 6 Slices bacon
- 6 Fluid Ounce pineapple juice
- 1 Teaspoon garlic, minced
- 2 Tablespoon honey

Directions:

1.   Remove the membrane from the bone side of the ribs and apply the salt, pepper and rub to that side. Flip the ribs over and season the meat side.

2.   Supply your smoker with wood pellets and follow the start-up procedure. Preheat the grill, with the lid closed, to 350° F.

3.   While the grill heats up, cook the bacon in a frying pan. As the bacon is cooking, pour the pineapple juice, garlic and honey into an oven safe pot.

4.   Remove the bacon from the grease and let the pan and bacon fat cool down. After the pan has cooled for a while, pour the bacon grease in with the pineapple juice, garlic and honey and stir to combine.

5.   Place the ribs and the pot on the grill and close the lid. After an hour, the slurry will have reduced down a bit and can be applied to the ribs. Slather the ribs with the reduction every 15 minutes. When the bones peek out about a quarter to a third of an inch, the ribs are done which is about 2 hours and 15 minutes. Grill: 350 °F

6.   For fall off the bone ribs, go another 30-45 minutes, continuing to glaze every 15 minutes. Grill: 350 °F

7.   The sweet and savory of the reduction will temper the heat of the spicy rub forming an outstanding and complex blend of flavors. Enjoy!

Beer Braised Garlic Bbq Pork Butt

Servings: 6-8

Cooking Time: 300 Minutes

Ingredients:

- One 12Oz Bottle Dark Beer
- 1/2 Cup Brown Sugar
- 2 Tablespoons Granulated Garlic
- 4 Tablespoons Honey
- 1 Cup Ketchup
- 1 Tablespoon Olive Oil
- Pulled Pork Rub
- 1 Pork Butt, Boneless
- 2 Tablespoons Worcestershire Sauce
- 4 Tablespoons Yellow Mustard

Directions:

1.   Generously season the pork butt with Pulled Pork Rub, making sure to rub the seasoning in on all surfaces of roast. Place the pork onto a roasting rack inside a 9x13 pan.

2. Pour about half a bottle of dark beer into the bottom of the pan and save the remaining amount of beer, you'll need this later.

3. Supply your smoker with wood pellets and follow the start-up procedure. Preheat the grill, with the lid open, to high heat. If you're using a gas or charcoal, set it up for high direct heat. Place the pan in the center of the grill and grill for 30 minutes until the pork roast is dark in color and charred in some spots.

4. Remove the pork from the grill and decrease the temperature of the grill to 325°F. Set aside and began to make the BBQ sauce.

5. In a medium sized bowl, add ketchup, brown sugar, yellow mustard, honey, Worcestershire, granulated garlic, half bottle of dark beer, and finally 1 tbsp of Pulled Pork Rub. Mix together thoroughly.

6. Take the sauce and pour it over the roast, cover with aluminum foil.

7. Cook the roast for 4 - 6 hours or until the meat is falling apart tender and the bone easily comes away from the meat and reaches an internal temperature of 200°F. Remove the pork from the grill and allow it to rest for 10-15 minutes.

8. Shred the pork with meat claws or forks, discarding any fat or gristle. Toss the shredded pork with the barbecue sauce and serve immediately.

Grilled Bacon Dog

Servings: 4
Cooking Time: 25 Minutes

Ingredients:
- 16 hot dogs
- 16 Slices Bacon, sliced
- 2 Vidalia onion, sliced
- 16 hot dog buns
- 'Que BBQ Sauce
- Velveeta cheese

Directions:
1. Supply your smoker with wood pellets and follow the start-up procedure. Preheat the grill, with the lid closed, to 375° F.

2. Wrap bacon strips around the hot dogs, and grill directly on the grill grate for 10 minutes each side. Grill onions at the same time as the hot dogs, and cook for 10 -15 minutes.

3. Open hot dog buns and spread Traeger 'Que sauce, the grilled hot dogs, cheese sauce and grilled onions. Top with vegetables. Serve, enjoy!

VEGETABLES RECIPES

Smoked Beet-pickled Eggs

Servings: 4

Cooking Time: 30 Minutes

Ingredients:

- 6 Eggs, hard boiled
- 1 Red Beets, scrubbed and trimmed
- 1 Cup apple cider vinegar
- 1 Cup Beet, juice
- 1/4 Onion, Sliced
- 1/3 Cup granulated sugar
- 3 Cardamom
- 1 star anise

Directions:

1. Supply your smoker with wood pellets and follow the start-up procedure. Preheat the grill, with the lid closed, to 275° F.

2. Place the peeled hard boiled eggs directly on the grill and smoke for 30 minutes. Grill: 275 °F

3. Put the smoked eggs in a quart size glass jar with the cooked/chopped beets in the bottom.

4. In a medium sauce pan, add the vinegar, beet juice, onion, sugar, cardamom and anise.

5. Bring to a boil and cook, uncovered, until sugar has dissolved and the onions are translucent (about 5 minutes).

6. Remove from the heat and let cool for a few minutes.

7. Pour the vinegar and onions mixture over the eggs and beets in the jar, covering the eggs completely.

8. Securely close with the jar lid. Refrigerate up to a month. Enjoy!

Baked Heirloom Tomato Tart

Servings: 4

Cooking Time: 45 Minutes

Ingredients:

- 1 Whole Puff Pastry Sheet
- 2 Pound heirloom tomatoes, various shapes and sizes
- 1/2 Tablespoon kosher salt
- 1/2 Cup Ricotta Cheese
- 5 Whole eggs
- 1 To Taste salt and pepper
- 1/2 Teaspoon thyme leaves
- 1/2 Teaspoon red pepper flakes
- 4 Sprig thyme

Directions:

1. Supply your smoker with wood pellets and follow the start-up procedure. Preheat the grill, with the lid closed, to 350° F.

2. Place the puff pastry on a parchment lined sheet tray, and make a cut ¾ of the way through the pastry, ½" from the edge.

3. Slice the tomatoes and season with salt. Place on a sheet tray lined with paper towels.

4. In a small bowl combine the ricotta, 4 of the eggs, salt, thyme leaves, red pepper flakes and black pepper. Whisk together until combined. Spread the ricotta mixture over the puff pastry, staying within ½" from the edge.

5. In a small bowl whisk the last egg. Brush the egg wash onto the exposed edges of the pastry.

6. Place the sheet tray directly on the grill grate and bake for 45 minutes, rotating half-way through. Grill: 350 °F

7. When the edges are browned and the moisture from the tomatoes has evaporated, remove from the grill and let cool 5-7 minutes before serving. Enjoy!

Grilled Corn On The Cob With Parmesan And Garlic

Servings: 6

Cooking Time: 30 Minutes

Ingredients:

- 4 Tablespoon butter, melted
- 2 Clove garlic, minced
- salt and pepper
- 8 ears fresh corn
- 1/2 Cup shaved Parmesan
- 1 Tablespoon chopped parsley

Directions:

1. Supply your smoker with wood pellets and follow the start-up procedure. Preheat the grill, with the lid closed, to 450° F.

2. Place butter, garlic, salt and pepper in a medium bowl and mix well.

3. Peel back corn husks and remove the silk. Rub corn with half of the garlic butter mixture.

4. Close husks and place directly on the grill grate. Cook for 25 to 30 minutes, turning occasionally until corn is tender. Grill: 450 ˚F

5. Remove from grill, peel and discard husks. Place corn on serving tray, drizzle with remaining butter and top with Parmesan and parsley.

Sicilian Stuffed Mushrooms

Servings: 6

Cooking Time: 25 Minutes

Ingredients:

- 12 Medium Fresh Mushrooms, about 1-1/2 inches in diameter
- 4 Ounce cream cheese, room temperature
- 1/4 Cup Parmesan cheese, grated
- 1/4 Cup shredded mozzarella cheese
- 8 Whole Pimento Stuffed Green Olives, chopped
- 3 Tablespoon Pepperoni, finely diced
- 1 1/2 Tablespoon Sun Dried Tomatoes, drained & minced
- 1/4 Teaspoon freshly ground black pepper

Directions:

1. Dampen a paper towel and wipe the outside of the mushrooms clean. Remove the stem. Using a small spoon, scoop out the inside of the mushroom leaving a shell.

2. Filling: In a small mixing bowl, beat together the cream cheese, Parmesan, and mozzarella. Stir in olives, pepperoni, tomatoes, basil, and pepper.

3. Mound the filling in the mushroom caps. Set each filled cap into the well of a muffin tin.

4. Supply your smoker with wood pellets and follow the start-up procedure. Preheat the grill, with the lid closed, to 350° F.

5. Arrange the muffin tin on the grill grate and bake the mushrooms for 25 to 30 minutes, or until the mushrooms are tender and the filling is beginning to brown.

6. Transfer to a serving plate or platter. Enjoy!

Sweet Potato Marshmallow Casserole

Servings: 6

Cooking Time: 60 Minutes

Ingredients:

- 5 Yams
- 1 1/2 Stick butter

- ➢ 1/2 Cup brown sugar
- ➢ 1 Teaspoon vanilla
- ➢ 1 Teaspoon kosher salt
- ➢ 1 Teaspoon cracked black pepper
- ➢ 1 Marshmallows, miniature
- ➢ 1/4 Unsalted Butter, Softened

Directions:

1. Supply your smoker with wood pellets and follow the start-up procedure. Preheat the grill, with the lid closed, to 375° F.

2. Pierce the skin of the yams with a fork a few times. Place on a baking sheet or foil tin inside the grill and let roast for 50 minutes or until extremely softened. Grill: 375 ℉

3. Remove yams from the grill and set aside until cool enough to handle. While the potatoes cool, with a stiff whisk, whip together 1/2 cup softened butter, the brown sugar, vanilla, salt and pepper.

4. Remove and discard skins from sweet potatoes and mash until smooth. Fold in the butter mixture and transfer to a cast iron pan.

5. Place cast iron on the grill and bake for 15-20 minutes. Remove from the grill, top with marshmallows and dot with remaining 1/4 cup butter.

6. Place back in the grill for 15 minutes until warm and the marshmallows are golden. Enjoy! Grill: 375 ℉

Grilled Cabbage Steaks With Warm Bacon Vinaigrette

Servings: 4

Cooking Time: 10 Minutes

Ingredients:

- ➢ 3 Strips thick-cut lean bacon, cut into 1/4 inch strips

- ➢ 1 Large shallot, minced
- ➢ 2 Tablespoon sherry vinegar
- ➢ 1 Tablespoon whole grain mustard
- ➢ 1 Teaspoon chopped thyme
- ➢ 2 Tablespoon olive oil, plus more as needed
- ➢ 1 Head green cabbage, cut into 3/4 inch thick slices (about 6 steaks)
- ➢ salt and pepper

Directions:

1. Supply your smoker with wood pellets and follow the start-up procedure. Preheat the grill, with the lid closed, to 450° F.

2. For the Vinaigrette: In a large skillet, cook the bacon in 2 tablespoons olive oil over medium-high heat until browned and crisp. Remove bacon from heat and stir in the shallot, vinegar, mustard and thyme then set aside.

3. Brush cabbage steaks with olive oil and season with salt and pepper. Place cabbage steaks directly on grill grate and grill for 5 minutes per side. Grill: 450 ℉

4. Remove cabbage steaks from grill and drizzle with bacon vinaigrette. Enjoy!

Portobello Marinated Mushroom

Servings: 2

Cooking Time: 15 Minutes

Ingredients:

- ➢ 1 Teaspoon chopped thyme
- ➢ 1 Teaspoon rosemary, chopped
- ➢ 1 Teaspoon Oregano, chopped
- ➢ 3 Tablespoon extra-virgin olive oil
- ➢ 1 To Taste Jacobsen Salt Co. Pure Kosher Sea Salt
- ➢ 1 To Taste pepper
- ➢ 6 Whole Portobello Mushroom
- ➢ 2 Whole russet potatoes

Directions:

1. Supply your smoker with wood pellets and follow the start-up procedure. Preheat the grill, with the lid closed, to 450° F.

2. Mix fresh herbs, olive oil, salt, and pepper together in a bowl. Rub over mushrooms. Grill both sides of mushrooms for approximately 2-3 minutes on each side. Grill: 450 ℉

3. Clean the potatoes and slice into long strips.

4. Heat the oil on the Traeger in a sauce pan; drop the potatoes in the hot oil and fry for 7-8 minutes. Let the potatoes cool slightly on a sheet pan. Enjoy! Grill: 450 ℉

Grilled Chili-lime Corn

Servings: 8
Cooking Time: 45 Minutes

Ingredients:

➢ 12 Corn, ears
➢ 1 Teaspoon chili powder
➢ 1/2 Teaspoon onion powder
➢ 1 Teaspoon   Leinenkugel's Summer Shandy Rub
➢ 2 lime, juiced
➢ 1 Tablespoon lime zest

Directions:

1. Soak the ears of corn, still in their husk, in water for 4 to 8 hours.

2. Supply your smoker with wood pellets and follow the start-up procedure. Preheat the grill, with the lid closed, to 350° F.

3. Place corn directly on grill grates. Turn corn every 15 minutes for 45 minutes total cooking time. Grill: 350 ℉

4. Combine chili powder, onion powder, Summer Shandy rub, lime juice, lime zest and butter in an oven safe dish and place in grill for

10 minutes. Remove corn and butter from the grill.

5. Pull corn husk back, but not off and remove corn silk. Using the corn husk as a handle, brush the corn with the melted chili-lime butter. Enjoy!

Spicy Asian Brussels Sprouts

Servings: 4
Cooking Time: 10 Minutes

Ingredients:

➢ 2 Cup fresh Brussels sprouts
➢ 2 Tablespoon vegetable oil
➢ 1 Tablespoon Asian BBQ Rub
➢ 1/4 Cup Thai sweet chile sauce

Directions:

1. Supply your smoker with wood pellets and follow the start-up procedure. Preheat the grill, with the lid closed, to 350° F.

2. Spread the halved brussel sprouts in a single layer on a lined cookie sheet. Drizzle with the oil and toss to coat.

3. Sprinkle the brussel sprouts evenly with an Asian BBQ rub and put the cookie sheet on the grill. Close the lid and cook for 7-8 minutes. Grill: 350 ℉

4. Toss the brussels sprouts in the Thai Chili Sauce and return to the grill for an additional 3-4 minutes, or until the sprouts are crisp-tender. Grill: 350 ℉

5. Serve immediately. Enjoy!

Baked Sweet Potato Casserole With Marshmallow Fluff

Servings: 6

Cooking Time: 60 Minutes

Ingredients:

- 3 Pound sweet potatoes
- 1/2 Cup milk
- 1 Cup brown sugar
- 3 eggs
- 4 Tablespoon butter
- 1/2 Teaspoon salt
- 3 egg white
- 1 Pinch salt
- 1 Pinch ground cinnamon

Directions:

1. Supply your smoker with wood pellets and follow the start-up procedure. Preheat the grill, with the lid closed, to 375° F.

2. Rinse, dry and pierce the sweet potatoes and place in grill whole. Cook for 45 minutes or until fork tender. Remove from grill and peel. Grill: 375 °F

3. Once peeled, mash the sweet potatoes in a large bowl with the milk, brown sugar, eggs, butter and salt. Place mashed potatoes in a baking dish and cook for 35 minutes. Grill: 375 °F

4. While the potatoes bake, make the fluff. Make a double boiler by bringing a small pot of water to a simmer, then placing the bowl of your stand mixer or another large stainless steel bowl atop the water.

5. Add the 3 egg whites, 2/3 cup brown sugar, a pinch of salt and a pinch of cinnamon to the bowl and whisk continuously until the sugar dissolves and the liquid is warm to the touch.

6. Transfer the bowl from the stovetop to your stand mixer and use the whisk attachment to whip the whites on medium-high speed until it turns glossy with stiff peaks, about 5-8 minutes.

7. Once the casserole has finished baking, use a rubber spatula to cover the sweet potato mixture with the fluff. Use the back of the spatula to create dramatic peaks.

8. Return to the grill for 5-7 minutes, or until the fluff starts to turn golden and the peaks are just shy of burnt. Remove from grill and enjoy!

Traeger Grilled Whole Corn

Servings: 4

Cooking Time: 25 Minutes

Ingredients:

- 3 green onions
- 6 Tablespoon butter, softened
- 1 Teaspoon chile powder
- 1 Teaspoon toasted sesame seeds
- 4 ears corn, in husk

Directions:

1. Supply your smoker with wood pellets and follow the start-up procedure. Preheat the grill, with the lid closed, to 325° F.

2. Place green onions directly on the grill grate and cook 15 minutes until lightly charred. Remove from grill and set aside.

3. Sesame-Chile Butter: Take butter out of fridge and let soften. Chop up charred green onions and add to butter along with chile powder and sesame seeds. Mash all ingredients together.

4. Grill corn, rotating occasionally, until husks are blackened (some will flake and fall off) and kernels are tender with some browned and charred spots, about 25 to 35 minutes. Grill: 325 °F

5. Let corn cool slightly, then shuck. Serve with the Sesame-Chile Butter. Enjoy

Smoked Mushrooms

Servings: 4
Cooking Time: 45 Minutes

Ingredients:
- Pound Mushrooms, fresh
- 1/2 Cup apple cider vinegar
- 1/2 Cup soy sauce
- 1 Teaspoon Blackened Saskatchewan Rub

Directions:
1. Clean mushrooms and place in a large Ziploc bag. Add apple cider vinegar, soy sauce and rub.
2. Mix well and allow to marinate in the refrigerator for at least 2 hours.
3. Supply your smoker with wood pellets and follow the start-up procedure. Preheat the grill, with the lid closed, to 350° F.
4. Place cast iron skillet inside grill for 20 minutes to warm up.
5. Add the mushrooms and marinade slowly into the cast iron skillet.
6. Cook uncovered for 15 minutes, then cover the skillet and cook another 30 minutes until mushrooms are tender. Grill: 350 °F
7. Remove skillet from grill and let mushrooms cool down for 5 minutes before serving. Enjoy!

Smoked Bbq Onion Brussels Sprout

Servings: 4
Cooking Time: 110 Minutes

Ingredients:
- 4 strip bacon
- 1 onion minced
- 2 cloves garlic minced
- 1 lb brussels sprouts stems trimmed and cut in half
- 1 tbsp BBQ Spice Blend
- 1/2 cup Apple Habanero Bar-B-Que Sauce (or other BBQ sauce)

Directions:
1. Supply your smoker with wood pellets and follow the start-up procedure. Preheat the grill, with the lid closed, to High heat. Place a cast iron skillet over the highest heat spot and cook the bacon until crisp.
2. Remove the bacon from pan and drain, reserving the bacon fat in the pan.
3. Reduce the heat on your smoker to 250°F.
4. Add the onions, garlic, and brussels to the pan and toss to coat in the bacon drippings. Sprinkle the BBQ spice blend over top.
5. Cover the lid and allow to smoke for 1 to 1 1/2 hours, until the sprouts are fork tender.
6. For the last 20 minutes of smoking, toss the brussels sprouts in half of the barbecue sauce.
7. Remove the sprouts from the smoker.
8. Chop the bacon and add it and the remaining barbecue sauce to the pan of sprouts, tossing to coat.
9. Serve hot.

Bacon Wrapped Corn On The Cob

Servings: 4
Cooking Time: 21 Minutes

Ingredients:
- 4 Whole Corn, ears
- 8 Slices bacon
- 1 Teaspoon freshly ground black pepper
- 1 Teaspoon chili powder
- 1 To Taste Parmesan cheese, grated

Directions:

1. Peel back the corn husks, remove silk strings and rinse corn under cold water.

2. Wrap 2 pieces of bacon around each ear of corn, securing with toothpicks.

3. Dust each ear of corn with some chili powder and cracked black pepper.

4. Supply your smoker with wood pellets and follow the start-up procedure. Preheat the grill, with the lid closed, to 375° F.

5. Place the ears of corn directly on the Traeger and grill for approximately 20 minutes or until the bacon is cooked crisp. Grill: 375 ℉

6. Take the corn off the Traeger. Carefully remove the toothpicks and season with a little more chili powder and a grating of parmesan cheese, if desired. Serve & enjoy!

Whole Roasted Cauliflower With Garlic Parmesan Butter

Servings: 4
Cooking Time: 45 Minutes

Ingredients:
- 1 Whole head cauliflower
- 1/4 Cup olive oil
- salt and pepper
- 1/2 Cup butter, melted
- 1/4 Cup shredded Parmesan cheese
- 2 Clove garlic, minced
- 1/2 Tablespoon chopped parsley

Directions:
1. Supply your smoker with wood pellets and follow the start-up procedure. Preheat the grill, with the lid closed, to 450° F.

2. Brush the cauliflower with olive oil and season liberally with salt and pepper.

3. Put cauliflower in a cast iron skillet, place directly on the grill grate and cook for 45 minutes until golden brown and the center is tender.

4. While the cauliflower is cooking, combine the melted butter, parmesan, garlic and parsley in a small bowl.

5. During the last 20 minutes of cooking, baste the cauliflower with the melted butter mixture.

6. Remove the cauliflower from the grill and top with extra parmesan and parsley if desired. Enjoy!

Smoked Parmesan Herb Popcorn

Servings: 2
Cooking Time: 15 Minutes

Ingredients:
- 4 Tablespoon butter
- 2 Teaspoon Italian Seasoning
- 1 Teaspoon garlic powder
- 1 Teaspoon salt
- 1/4 Cup popcorn kernels
- 1/2 Cup Parmesan cheese, grated

Directions:
1. Supply your smoker with wood pellets and follow the start-up procedure. Preheat the grill, with the lid closed, to 250° F.

2. In a small saucepan, melt the butter over medium heat. Add Italian seasoning, garlic powder, and salt and stir to combine. Remove from heat and set aside.

3. Add 1/4 cup of popcorn to a brown paper lunch bag. Fold the top of the bag over twice to close. Place the bag in the microwave and microwave on high for 1 to 2 minutes, or until there are about 5 seconds between pops. Open the bag with care and dump into a large mixing bowl.

4. Pour butter mixture of popcorn in a bowl and toss to combine. Dump popcorn onto a baking sheet and place in grill.

5. Smoke for 10 minutes; remove from grill. Toss with parmesan cheese to serve. Enjoy! Grill: 250 ˚F

Roasted Red Pepper White Bean Dip

Servings: 4
Cooking Time: 40 Minutes

Ingredients:
- 4 Whole garlic
- 4 Tablespoon extra-virgin olive oil
- 2 Bell Pepper, Red
- 3 Tablespoon Dill Weed, fresh
- 3 Tablespoon chopped flat-leaf parsley
- 2 Can cannellini beans, mashed
- 4 Teaspoon lemon juice
- 1 1/2 Teaspoon salt

Directions:
1. Roasting the garlic and red peppers:
2. Supply your smoker with wood pellets and follow the start-up procedure. Preheat the grill, with the lid closed, to 400° F.
3. Peel away the outside layers of the garlic husk. Cut off the top of the garlic bulb, exposing each of the individual cloves. Drizzle olive oil over the top of the head of garlic and rub it in. Wrap the garlic in foil, completely covering it. Put the head of garlic and the two red peppers (washed and dried) on the Traeger.
4. Roast the garlic for 25-30 minutes and the peppers for about 40 minutes. Rotate the peppers a quarter-turn every 10 minutes until the exterior is blistered and blackened. Grill: 400 ˚F

5. Pull the peppers off the grill and put them in a bowl. Cover the bowl with plastic wrap and leave them for 15 minutes. The steam will loosen the skins so that they slip off like a drumstick covered in barbecue sauce.
6. Peel off the pepper skin. Cut off the stems and scrape out the seeds and they're ready to use.
7. As for the garlic, let it cool and then pull out the individual cloves as needed.
8. The dip:
9. In a blender put the roasted red peppers, 4 cloves of roasted garlic, dill, parsley, drained and rinsed beans, olive oil, lemon juice and salt.
10. Blend until the dip is smooth and creamy. You may need to scrape down the sides of the blender a couple of times. If it's having difficulty blending or looks too thick add more olive oil or lemon juice. (Add more lemon juice if it tastes like it needs more acid or brightness.) Enjoy!

Smoked Pickled Green Beans

Servings: 4
Cooking Time: 45 Minutes

Ingredients:
- 1 Pound Green Beans, blanched
- 1/2 Cup salt
- 1/2 Cup sugar
- 1 Tablespoon red pepper flakes
- 2 Cup white wine vinegar
- 2 Cup ice water

Directions:
1. Supply your smoker with wood pellets and follow the start-up procedure. Preheat the grill, with the lid closed, to 180° F.
2. Place the blanched green beans on a mesh grill mat and place mat directly on the grill grate. Smoke the green beans for 30-45 minutes until

they've picked up the desired amount of smoke. Remove from grill and set aside until the brine is ready. Grill: 180 ˚F

3. In a medium sized saucepan, bring all remaining ingredients, except ice water, to a boil over medium high heat on the stove. Simmer for 5-10 minutes then remove from heat and steep 20 minutes more. Pour brine over ice water to cool.

4. Once brine has cooled, pour over the green beans and weigh them down with a few plates to ensure they are completely submerged. Let sit 24 hours before use. Enjoy!

Baked Sweet Potatoes

Servings: 8
Cooking Time: 60 Minutes

Ingredients:
- 1 Cup butter, softened
- 1/4 Cup pure maple syrup
- 1/2 Teaspoon ground cinnamon
- 8 Medium sweet potatoes

Directions:
1. Make the Maple-Cinnamon Butter: In a mixing bowl, combine the butter, maple syrup, and cinnamon and whip with a wooden spoon. (Alternatively, blend the ingredients using a hand-held mixer or a stand mixer.) Transfer to a small bowl, cover, and chill until serving time.
2. Supply your smoker with wood pellets and follow the start-up procedure. Preheat the grill, with the lid closed, to 375° F. Arrange the sweet potatoes on the grill grate and bake until soft, 1 to 1-1/2 hours, depending on the size of the potatoes. Make a slit in the side of each, and squeeze the ends gently to fluff.
3. Serve hot with the Maple-Cinnamon Butter. Enjoy!

Baked Sweet And Savory Yams By Bennie Kendrick

Servings: 6
Cooking Time: 60 Minutes

Ingredients:
- 3 Medium Yams
- 3 Tablespoon extra-virgin olive oil
- honey
- Goat Cheese
- 1/2 Cup brown sugar
- 1/2 Cup Pecans, pieces

Directions:
1. Supply your smoker with wood pellets and follow the start-up procedure. Preheat the grill, with the lid closed, to 350° F.
2. While Traeger comes to temperature, wash yams and poke a few holes all over. Wrap yams in foil.
3. Bake for 45-60 minutes or until knife tender. You don't want to overcook and get the yams too soft because you want to be able to cut each yam into rounds.
4. Once yams have cooled to the touch, cut each into 1/4" rounds. Lightly coat each round with oil olive and place on sheet tray.
5. Sprinkle each top with brown sugar. Using a teaspoon, place desired amount of goat cheese on each round. Next top with chopped pecans. Finally, drizzle Bee Local honey over each round.
6. Based on how sweet you like your yams, you can add more brown sugar and honey.
7. After complete, place your sheet tray back in the grill and cook, lid closed, for another 20 minutes. Enjoy!

Roasted Mashed Potatoes

Servings: 8

Cooking Time: 40 Minutes

Ingredients:
- 5 Pound Yukon Gold potatoes
- 1 1/2 Stick butter, softened
- 1 1/2 Cup heavy whipping cream, room temperature
- kosher salt
- white pepper

Directions:

1. Supply your smoker with wood pellets and follow the start-up procedure. Preheat the grill, with the lid closed, to 300° F.

2. Peel and cut potatoes into 1/2 inch cubes. Place the potatoes in a shallow baking dish with 1/2 cup water and cover. Bake until tender, about 40 minutes. Grill: 300 ℉

3. In a medium saucepan, combine cream and butter. Cook over medium heat until butter is melted.

4. Remove potatoes from the grill and drain water.

5. Transfer potatoes to a bowl and mash using a potato masher. Gradually add in cream and butter mixture and mix using the masher. Be careful not to overwork or the potatoes will becomes gluey. Season with salt and pepper to taste. Enjoy!

Baked Bacon Green Bean Casserole

Servings: 6

Cooking Time: 50 Minutes

Ingredients:
- 1 1/2 Pound Green Beans, fresh
- 1 Can cream of mushroom soup
- 1/2 Cup milk
- 1/2 Teaspoon Worcestershire sauce
- 1/2 Teaspoon black pepper
- 2/3 Cup French's Original Crispy Fried Onions
- 8 Slices bacon
- 1/4 Cup red bell pepper, diced
- 2/3 French's Original Crispy Fried Onions

Directions:

1. In a mixing bowl, combine beans, soup, milk, Worcestershire sauce, black pepper, 2/3 cup of the onions, 6 of the slices of crumbled bacon, and red bell pepper. Transfer to a 1-1/2 quart casserole dish.

2. Supply your smoker with wood pellets and follow the start-up procedure. Preheat the grill, with the lid closed, to 350° F.

3. Cook casserole until the filling is hot and bubbling, 35 to 40 minutes. Grill: 350 ℉

4. Top with remaining onions and the last 2 slices of crumbled bacon and cook for 5 to 10 minutes more, or until the onions are crisp and beginning to brown. Serve, enjoy! Grill: 350 ℉

Roasted Tomatoes

Servings: 2

Cooking Time: 180 Minutes

Ingredients:
- 3 Large ripe tomatoes
- 1/2 Tablespoon kosher salt
- 1 Teaspoon coarse ground black pepper
- 1/4 Teaspoon sugar
- 1/4 Teaspoon thyme or basil
- olive oil

Directions:

1. Line a rimmed baking sheet with parchment paper.

2. Supply your smoker with wood pellets and follow the start-up procedure. Preheat the grill, with the lid closed, to 225° F.

3. Remove the stem end from each tomato and cut the tomatoes into 1/2 inch thick slices.

4. Combine the salt, pepper, sugar and thyme or basil in a small bowl and mix.

5. Pour olive oil into the well of a dinner plate.

6. Dip one side of each tomato slice in the olive oil and arrange on the baking sheet. Dust the tomato slices with the seasoning mixture.

7. Arrange the pan directly on the grill grate and roast the tomatoes until the juices stop running and the edges have contracted, about 3 hours. Remove from grill and enjoy!

Baked Breakfast Mini Quiches

Servings: 8
Cooking Time: 15 Minutes

Ingredients:

- cooking spray
- 1 Tablespoon extra-virgin olive oil
- 1/2 yellow onion, diced
- 3 Cup Spinach, fresh
- 10 eggs
- 4 Ounce shredded cheddar, mozzarella or Swiss cheese
- 1/4 Cup fresh basil
- 1 Teaspoon kosher salt
- 1/2 Teaspoon black pepper

Directions:

1. Spray a 12-cup muffin tin generously with cooking spray.

2. In a small skillet over medium heat, warm the oil. Add the onion and cook, stirring frequently, until softened, about 7 minutes. Add the spinach and cook until wilted, about 1 minute longer.

3. Transfer to a cutting board to cool, then chop the mixture so the spinach if broken up a little.

4. Supply your smoker with wood pellets and follow the start-up procedure. Preheat the grill, with the lid closed, to 350° F.

5. In a large bowl, whisk the eggs until frothy. Add the cooled onions and spinach, cheese, basil, 1 tsp salt and 1/2 tsp pepper. Stir to combine. Divide egg mixture evenly among the muffin cups.

6. Place tray on the grill and bake until the eggs have puffed up, are set, and are beginning to brown, about 18 to 20 minutes. Grill: 350 °F

7. Serve immediately, or allow to cool on a wire rack, then refrigerate in an air tight container for up to 4 days. Enjoy!

Grilled Broccoli Rabe

Servings: 4
Cooking Time: 10 Minutes

Ingredients:

- 4 Tablespoon extra-virgin olive oil
- 4 Bunch broccoli rabe or broccolini
- kosher salt
- 1 lemon, halved

Directions:

1. Supply your smoker with wood pellets and follow the start-up procedure. Preheat the grill, with the lid closed, to 450° F.

2. On a platter or in a mixing bowl, drizzle the olive oil over the broccoli rabe. Use your hands to mix thoroughly, coating the vegetables evenly with the oil. Season with sea salt.

3. Place the broccoli rabe in one layer directly on the lowest grill grate. Close the lid and cook for 5 to 10 minutes. You want there to be some color and slight char on the first side. Flip and cook for a few more minutes. Grill: 450 °F

4. Transfer the broccoli rabe to a serving platter and squeeze the juice of half a lemon evenly over the top.

5. Serve with more lemon wedges on the side. Enjoy!

Smoked Jalapeño Poppers

Servings: 4

Cooking Time: 60 Minutes

Ingredients:

- ➢ 12 Medium jalapeño
- ➢ 6 Slices bacon, cut in half
- ➢ 8 Ounce cream cheese
- ➢ 2 Tablespoon Pork & Poultry Rub
- ➢ 1 Cup grated cheese

Directions:

1. Supply your smoker with wood pellets and follow the start-up procedure. Preheat the grill, with the lid closed, to 180° F. For optimal flavor, use Super Smoke if available.

2. Slice the jalapeños in half lengthwise. Scrape out any seeds and ribs with a small spoon or paring knife. Mix softened cream cheese with Traeger Pork & Poultry rub and grated cheese. Spoon mixture onto each jalapeño half. Wrap with bacon and secure with a toothpick.

3. Place the jalapeños on a rimmed baking sheet. Place on grill and smoke for 30 minutes. Grill: 180 ˚F

4. Increase the grill temperature to 375˚F and cook an additional 30 minutes or until bacon is cooked to desired doneness. Serve warm, enjoy! Grill: 375 ˚F

POULTRY RECIPES

Bacon Wrapped Turkey Legs

Servings: 8

Cooking Time: 180 Minutes

Ingredients:

- 1 Gallon water
- 1/4 Cup Rub
- 3 Cup Morton Tender Quick Home Meat Cure
- 1/2 Cup brown sugar
- 6 Whole black peppercorns
- 2 Whole bay leaves
- 8 (1-1/2 lb each) turkey legs
- 8 Slices bacon

Directions:

1. Plan ahead, these turkey legs brine overnight. In a large stockpot, combine one gallon of water, Traeger Rub, curing salt, brown sugar, peppercorns and bay leaves.

2. Bring to a boil over high heat to dissolve the salt and sugar granules. Take off of the heat and add in 1/2 gallon of water and ice. Make sure the brine is at least to room temperature, if not colder. (You may need to refrigerate the brine for an hour or so.)

3. Add the turkey legs making sure they are completely submerged in the brine.

4. After 24 hours, drain the turkey legs and discard the brine. Rinse the brine off the legs with cold water, then dry thoroughly with paper towels.

5. Supply your smoker with wood pellets and follow the start-up procedure. Preheat the grill, with the lid closed, to 250° F.

6. Lay the turkey legs directly on the grill grate.

7. After 2-1/2 hours, wrap a piece of bacon around each leg and finish cooking them for the last 30 to 40 minutes. Grill: 250 ℉

8. The total cooking time for the legs will be 3 hours, or until the internal temperature reaches 165°F on an instant-read meat thermometer. Serve and enjoy! Grill: 250 ℉ Probe: 165 ℉

Grilled Honey Chicken Kabobs

Servings: 4

Cooking Time: 14 Minutes

Ingredients:

- 1 pound boneless skinless chicken breasts (cut into 1 inch pieces)
- 1/4 cup olive oil
- 1/3 cup soy sauce
- 1/4 cup honey
- 1 teaspoon minced garlic
- salt and pepper to taste
- 1 red bell pepper (cut into 1 inch pieces)
- 1 yellow bell pepper (cut into 1 inch pieces)
- 2 small zucchini (cut into 1 inch slices)
- 1 red onion (cut into 1 inch pieces)
- 1 tablespoon chopped parsley

Directions:

1. In a large bowl combine the olive oil, soy sauce, honey, garlic and salt and pepper, and whisk.

2. Add the chicken, bell peppers, zucchini and red onion to the bowl, tossing to thoroughly coat.

3. Cover and refrigerate for 1 to 8 hours.

4. Soak wooden skewers in cold water for at least 30 minutes. Supply your smoker with wood pellets and follow the start-up procedure. Preheat the grill, with the lid closed, to high heat.

5. Thread the chicken and vegetables onto the skewers.

6. Cook for 5-7 minutes on each side or until chicken is cooked through.

7. To serve, sprinkle with parsley. Enjoy!

Grilled Honey Chicken Wings

Servings: 4 - 8

Cooking Time: 30 Minutes

Ingredients:

- 2 Chipotles Chopped In Adobo
- 1 Apple Cider Vinegar
- 2 Tablespoons Balsamic Vinegar
- ¼ Cup Brown Sugar
- 2 ½ Lbs Chicken Wings, Trimmed And Patted Dry
- ¼ Cup Honey
- ½ Cup Ketchup
- ¼ Cup Adobo Sauce
- 2 Tablespoons Sweet Rib Rub
- 2 Teaspoons Worcestershire Sauce

Directions:

1. Supply your smoker with wood pellets and follow the start-up procedure. Preheat the grill, with the lid open, to 350° F. If you're using a charcoal or gas grill, set up the grill for medium high heat.

2. In a large bowl, whisk together the apple cider vinegar, ketchup, brown sugar, honey, chopped chipotle peppers with adobo sauce, balsamic vinegar, Worcestershire sauce, and Sweet Rib Rub. Whisk the glaze until it's well combined.

3. Add the wings to the glaze and place the bowl in the refrigerator. Marinade the chicken wings for up to 12 hours. Once the wings have finished marinating, remove the chicken wings from the marinade and place the chicken wings onto the wing rack.

4. Once all the wings have been placed on the wing rack, place the wing rack on the grill. Insert a temperature probe into the thickest part into one of the wings and grill the wings for 5 minutes, and then rotate the rack 180° and grill for another 5 minutes. Remove the wings once they have an internal temperature of 165°F and the juice from the chicken runs clear.

5. Remove the wings from the grill and serve immediately.

Chile Cilantro Lime Chicken Wings

Servings: 4

Cooking Time: 20 Minutes

Ingredients:

- 1 Tsp Ancho Chili Powder
- 2 Tsp Blackened Sriracha Rub Seasoning
- 2 Lbs Chicken Wings, Split
- 2 Tbsp Cilantro, Chopped, Divided
- 1 Tsp Cumin
- 1 Lime, Zest & Juice
- 1 1/2 Tbsp Olive Oil

Directions:

1. In a medium bowl, combine 1 tablespoon of cilantro, lime juice and zest, olive oil, Blackened Sriracha, ancho chili powder, and cumin.

2. Place chicken wings in a resealable gallon bag and add cilantro mixture. Transfer to the refrigerator and marinate for 1 hour, turning occasionally.

3. Supply your smoker with wood pellets and follow the start-up procedure. Preheat the grill, with the lid closed, to 350° F. If using a gas or charcoal grill, set it up for medium heat.

4. Remove chicken wings from the marinade and place on the grill over indirect heat. Grill for 15 to 18 minutes, turning and rotating every 3 to 5 minutes.

5. Remove chicken wings from the grill, garnish with remaining cilantro, and serve warm.

Buffalo Chicken Wings

Servings: 4
Cooking Time: 20 Minutes

Ingredients:
- 1 1/2 Tbsp Apple Cider Vinegar
- 1/2 Cup Butter, Unsalted, Cubed
- 1/4 Tsp Cayenne Pepper
- 3 Lbs Chicken Wings, Split
- 2 Tsp Chives, Minced (Garnish)
- 1/8 Tsp Garlic, Granulated
- 2/3 Cup Hot Pepper Sauce
- 1 Tbsp Ranch Seasoning
- To Taste, Sweet Heat Rub
- 1/2 Tsp Sweet Heat Rub (For Sauce)
- 1/4 Tsp Worcestershire Sauce

Directions:
1. Supply your smoker with wood pellets and follow the start-up procedure. Preheat the grill, with the lid open, to 425° F. If using a gas or charcoal grill, set it up for medium-high heat.

2. Place chicken wings in a large mixing bowl. Season with Sweet Heat.

3. Prepare sauce: Set a small cast iron pan or saucepan on the grill. Add the hot pepper sauce, apple cider vinegar, Worcestershire sauce, Sweet Heat, cayenne, and granulated garlic to the skillet, and whisk to combine. When the sauce begins to bubble, remove the skillet from the grill and whisk in butter. Transfer the sauce to a mason jar.

4. Combine 1 cup of the buffalo sauce with ranch seasoning. Set aside.

5. Place wings on the grill and cook for 20 minutes, flipping and rotating every 3 to 5 minutes.

6. Remove wings from the grill when an internal temperature of 165° F is reached. Transfer to a mixing bowl, then pour sauce over. Toss to evenly coat. Garnish with fresh chives and serve warm.

Crispy Spiced Chicken Wings

Servings: 10
Cooking Time: 75 Minutes

Ingredients:
- 5 pounds of chicken wings (flats and drumettes)
- 2 1/2 Tablespoons baking powder
- 1 teaspoon salt

Directions:
1. Dry your chicken wings thoroughly on all sides with a paper towel. Place them in a zip-top bag.

2. Add the baking powder and salt to the wings, close the bag, and toss to coat evenly.

3. Supply your smoker with wood pellets and follow the start-up procedure. Preheat the grill, with the lid closed, to 250° F, using your favorite wood. Place the wings directly on the grill grates, close the lid, and smoke for 30 minutes.

4. Increase the heat in your smoker to 425 degrees F and continue cooking for 45 more minutes, or until the internal temperature of the wing reads 175 degrees F. You can rotate or flip the wings as needed to maintain even cooking and avoid any hot spots on the grill.

5. Remove the wing from the grill and serve. You can serve plain, toss in your favorite BBQ seasoning, or hot sauce.

Oktoberfest Pretzel Mustard Chicken

Servings: 4
Cooking Time: 25 Minutes

Ingredients:
- 1/4 Pound pretzel sticks
- 3 Tablespoon Dijon mustard
- 3 Tablespoon apple cider or brown ale
- 1 Tablespoon honey
- 1 1/2 Teaspoon fresh thyme, plus more for garnish
- 4 boneless, skinless chicken breasts

Directions:
1. Pulse the pretzel sticks in a food processor or crush by hand in a resealable bag until they've turned into a powder the texture of panko breadcrumbs.
2. Transfer the crumbs to a wide, shallow bowl.
3. In separate shallow bowl, whisk mustard, beer or cider, honey and thyme together.
4. Spray a wire rack with cooking spray and place atop a sheet tray. Dip each chicken breast in the mustard mixture, then dredge in the pretzel crumbs to coat evenly and place on the wire rack. Spray the top of each chicken breast lightly with cooking spray.
5. Supply your smoker with wood pellets and follow the start-up procedure. Preheat the grill, with the lid closed, to 375° F.
6. Place the pan on the Traeger and bake for about 20 to 25 minutes, until the chicken breasts are fully cooked and register 165°F on an instant-read thermometer. Grill: 375 °F Probe: 165 °F

7. Let chicken rest for 5 minutes. Garnish with fresh thyme if desired. Enjoy!

Wild West Wings

Servings: 4
Cooking Time: 60 Minutes

Ingredients:
- 2 pounds chicken wings
- 2 tablespoons extra-virgin olive oil
- 2 packages ranch dressing mix (such as Hidden Valley brand)
- ¼ cup prepared ranch dressing (optional)

Directions:
1. Supply your smoker with wood pellets and follow the start-up procedure. Preheat, with the lid closed, to 350°F.
2. Place the chicken wings in a large bowl and toss with the olive oil and ranch dressing mix.
3. Arrange the wings directly on the grill, or line the grill with aluminum foil for easy cleanup, close the lid, and smoke for 25 minutes.
4. Flip and smoke for 20 to 35 minutes more, or until a meat thermometer inserted in the thickest part of the wings reads 165°F and the wings are crispy. (Note: The wings will likely be done after 45 minutes, but an extra 10 to 15 minutes makes them crispy without drying the meat.)
5. Serve warm with ranch dressing (if using).

Savory Smoked Turkey Legs

Servings: 4
Cooking Time: 150 Minutes

Ingredients:
- 1 Cup Chicken Stock
- 2 Tbsp Blackened Sriracha Rub
- 4 Turkey Legs (Drumsticks)

Directions:

1. Fire up your   pellet grill on SMOKE mode. With the lid open, let it run for 10 minutes.

2. Supply your smoker with wood pellets and follow the start-up procedure. Preheat the grill, with the lid closed, to 225° F. If using a gas or charcoal grill, set it up for low, indirect heat.

3. Combine turkey stock with 2 teaspoons of Blackened Sriracha Rub.

4. Place turkey legs on a sheet tray, then inject each with seasoned stock. Season the outside of the legs with remaining Blackened Sriracha.

5. Place turkey legs directly on the grate of the smoking cabinet, and cook for 1 ½ hours.

6. Increase temperature to 325°F, then transfer turkey legs to the bottom grill and cook for another 45 to 60 minutes, until the internal temperature reaches 170°F.

7. Remove turkey from the grill, allow to rest for 10 minutes, then serve warm.

Smoked Wings

Servings: 6
Cooking Time: 50 Minutes

Ingredients:

➢ 24 chicken wings, flats and drumettes separated
➢ 12 Ounce Italian dressing
➢ 3 Ounce Chicken Rub
➢ 5 Ounce 'Que BBQ Sauce
➢ 3 Ounce chili sauce

Directions:

1. Wash all wings and place into resealable bag. Add Italian dressing to the resealable bag containing the wings. Place in refrigerator and allow to marinate for 6 to 12 hours.

2. Supply your smoker with wood pellets and follow the start-up procedure. Preheat the grill, with the lid closed, to 225° F.

3. Remove wings from marinade and shake off excess marinade. Season all sides of the wings with Traeger Chicken Rub and let sit for 15 minutes before putting wings on the Traeger.

4. In a small bowl, combine the BBQ and chili sauces. Set aside.

5. Cook wings to an internal temperature of 160°F. Remove the wings and toss in chili barbecue sauce. Grill: 225 °F Probe: 160 °F

6. Increase the grill temperature to 375°F and preheat. Once at temperature, place the wings on the Traeger and sear both sides until the internal temperature reaches 165°F. Grill: 375 °F Probe: 165 °F

7. Remove the wings from grill and let rest for 5 minutes. Serve with your favorite side wing dressing or sauce. Enjoy!

Smoked Turkey Breast

Servings: 2-4
Cooking Time: 120 Minutes

Ingredients:

➢ 1 (3-pound) turkey breast
➢ Salt
➢ Freshly ground black pepper
➢ 1 teaspoon garlic powder

Directions:

1. Supply your smoker with wood pellets and follow the start-up procedure. Preheat the grill, with the lid closed, to 180°F.

2. Season the turkey breast all over with salt, pepper, and garlic powder.

3. Place the breast directly on the grill grate and smoke for 1 hour.

4. Increase the grill's temperature to 350°F and continue to cook until the turkey's internal temperature reaches 170°F. Remove the breast from the grill and serve immediately.

Loaded Chicken Fries

Servings: 4
Cooking Time: 20 Minutes

Ingredients:
- 8 Slices Bacon, Cooked And Diced
- 1 12 Oz Bag Cheese, Shredded
- 1 Bag Fries, Frozen
- 2 Tablespoons Green Onions, Diced
- ¼ Cup White Barbecue Sauce

Directions:
1. Supply your smoker with wood pellets and follow the start-up procedure. Preheat the grill, with the lid open, to 400° F.
2. Bake the fries on the baking sheet in your according to the manufacturer's instructions. Once the fries are done, remove them from the grill and reduce the temperature to 350°F.
3. Top the fries with the cheese, chicken and bacon. Place the fries back on the grill and cook for another 5-7 minutes, or until the chicken is warmed through and the cheese is melted. Remove the fries from the grill.
4. Top the fries with the white barbecue sauce and green onions and serve immediately.

Jamaican Jerk Chicken Quarters

Servings: 4
Cooking Time: 120 Minutes

Ingredients:
- 4 chicken leg quarters, scored
- ¼ cup canola oil
- ½ cup Jamaican Jerk Paste
- 1 tablespoon whole allspice (pimento) berries

Directions:
1. Supply your smoker with wood pellets and follow the start-up procedure. Preheat, with the lid closed, to 275°F.
2. Brush the chicken with canola oil, then brush 6 tablespoons of the Jerk paste on and under the skin. Reserve the remaining 2 tablespoons of paste for basting.
3. Throw the whole allspice berries in with the wood pellets for added smoke flavor.
4. Arrange the chicken on the grill, close the lid, and smoke for 1 hour to 1 hour 30 minutes, or until a meat thermometer inserted in the thickest part of the thigh reads 165°F.
5. Let the meat rest for 5 minutes and baste with the reserved jerk paste prior to serving.

Smo-fried Chicken

Servings: 4-6
Cooking Time: 55 Minutes

Ingredients:
- 1 egg, beaten
- ½ cup milk
- 1 cup all-purpose flour
- 2 tablespoons salt
- 1 tablespoon freshly ground black pepper
- 2 teaspoons freshly ground white pepper
- 2 teaspoons cayenne pepper
- 2 teaspoons garlic powder
- 2 teaspoons onion powder
- 1 teaspoon smoked paprika
- 8 tablespoons (1 stick) unsalted butter, melted
- 1 whole chicken, cut up into pieces

Directions:

1. Supply your smoker with wood pellets and follow the start-up procedure. Preheat, with the lid closed, to 375°F.

2. In a medium bowl, combine the beaten egg with the milk and set aside.

3. In a separate medium bowl, stir together the flour, salt, black pepper, white pepper, cayenne, garlic powder, onion powder, and smoked paprika.

4. Line the bottom and sides of a high-sided metal baking pan with aluminum foil to ease cleanup.

5. Pour the melted butter into the prepared pan.

6. Dip the chicken pieces one at a time in the egg mixture, and then coat well with the seasoned flour. Transfer to the baking pan.

7. Smoke the chicken in the pan of butter ("smo-fry") on the grill, with the lid closed, for 25 minutes, then reduce the heat to 325°F and turn the chicken pieces over.

8. Continue smoking with the lid closed for about 30 minutes, or until a meat thermometer inserted in the thickest part of each chicken piece reads 165°F.

9. Serve immediately.

Smoked Bourbon & Orange Brined Turkey

Servings: 8
Cooking Time: 180 Minutes

Ingredients:
- 1 Orange Brine and Turkey Rub Kit
- 4 Quart water
- 1 Cup bourbon
- 1 (12-14 lb) turkey, fresh or thawed
- 1 Tablespoon butter, melted
- 1 Tablespoon Grand Mariner or other orange-flavored liquor

Directions:

1. Mix Orange Brine seasoning (from Traeger Orange Brine & Turkey Rub Kit) with one quart of water. Boil for 5 minutes. Remove from heat, add 3 quarts of cold water and bourbon. Refrigerate until completely cooled.

2. Place turkey breast side down in a large container. Pour cooled brine mix over bird. Add cold water until bird is submerged. Refrigerate for 24 hours.

3. Remove turkey and discard brine. Blot turkey dry with paper towels.

4. Combine butter and Grand Marnier and coat outside of turkey. Season outside of turkey with Traeger Turkey Rub (from Orange Brine & Turkey Rub Kit).

5. Supply your smoker with wood pellets and follow the start-up procedure. Preheat the grill, with the lid closed, to 225° F.

6. Smoke turkey, breast up, for 2 hours. Grill: 225 °F

7. Increase grill temperature to 350°F and roast turkey until the internal temperature of the thickest part of the thigh reaches 165F, 2 to 3 hours, depending on size of turkey. Grill: 350 °F Probe: 165 °F

8. Let rest 20 to 30 minutes before serving. Enjoy!

Smoked Quarters

Servings: 2-4
Cooking Time: 120 Minutes

Ingredients:
- 4 chicken quarters
- 2 tablespoons olive oil
- 1 batch Chicken Rub
- 2 tablespoons butter

Directions:

1. Supply your smoker with wood pellets and follow the start-up procedure. Preheat the grill, with the lid closed, to 180°F.
2. Coat the chicken quarters all over with olive oil and season them with the rub. Using your hands, work the rub into the meat.
3. Place the quarters directly on the grill grate and smoke for 1½ hours.
4. Baste the quarters with the butter and increase the grill's temperature to 375°F. Continue to cook until the chicken's internal temperature reaches 170°F.
5. Remove the quarters from the grill and let them rest for 10 minutes before serving.

Savory Smoked Chicken Breasts

Servings: 2
Cooking Time: 30 Minutes

Ingredients:

➢ 1 lb Boneless Skinless Chicken Breasts
➢ 2-3 Tbsp BBQ Chicken Rub

Directions:

1. Supply your smoker with wood pellets and follow the start-up procedure. Preheat the grill, with the lid closed, to 250° F.
2. Pound chicken breasts flat, about 1/2" thick. Rub the dry rub all over chicken breasts.
3. Place chicken breasts on the grill grate. Close pellet grill lid and cook at 250 °F for about 30 minutes or until the chicken reaches an internal temperature of 165 °F.
4. Remove from pellet grill and let rest 5-10 minutes.

Smoke Roasted Chicken With Herb Butter

Servings: 4
Cooking Time: 60 Minutes

Ingredients:

➢ 8 Tablespoon butter, room temperature
➢ 1 Scallions, minced
➢ 1 Clove garlic, minced
➢ 2 Tablespoon Fresh Herbs (Thyme, Rosemary, Oregano, Basil, Sage or Parsley, Minced)
➢ 1 1/2 Tablespoon Chicken Rub
➢ 1/2 Tablespoon fresh lemon juice
➢ 1 (4 to 4-1/2 lb) chicken
➢ Chicken Rub

Directions:

1. In a small bowl, combine butter, scallions, garlic, minced fresh herbs, Traeger Chicken Rub and lemon juice. Blend well with a wooden spoon.
2. Remove any giblets from the cavity of the chicken. Wash the chicken inside and out with cold running water. Dry thoroughly with paper towels.
3. Sprinkle a generous amount of Traeger Chicken Rub into the cavity of the chicken.
4. Gently loosen the skin around the chicken breast and slide in a few tablespoons of the herb butter and cover evenly. Smear the outside of the chicken with the remaining herb butter.
5. Tuck the chicken wings behind the back. Tie the legs together with butcher's twine.
6. Sprinkle the outside of the chicken with more Traeger Chicken Rub and insert sprigs of fresh herbs into the cavity of the chicken if desired.

7. Supply your smoker with wood pellets and follow the start-up procedure. Preheat the grill, with the lid closed, to 400° F.

8. When grill is hot, place chicken directly on the grill grate, breast side up. Cook for 1 to 1-1/4 hours or until the internal temperature registers 165°F. If the chicken is browning too quickly, loosely cover the breast and legs with foil and continue to cook. Grill: 400 °F Probe: 165 °F

9. Remove from the grill and let rest 15 minutes at room temperature before carving. Serve. Enjoy!

Smoked Honey Chicken Drumsticks

Servings: 4

Cooking Time: 30 Minutes

Ingredients:
- 1/2 Cup Apple Cider Vinegar
- 12 Chicken Drumsticks
- 2 Tablespoons Dijon Mustard
- 1/4 Cup Honey
- 1/4 Cup Ketchup
- 1 Tablespoon Sweet Heat Rub
- 1/2 Cup Soy Sauce

Directions:

1. Supply your smoker with wood pellets and follow the start-up procedure. Preheat the grill, with the lid open, to 225° F. Remove the wings from the marinade and place the drumsticks into the Buffalo Wing Rack.

2. Smoke for 60 minutes, or until a thermometer inserted into the thickest part of the drumstick registers at 170°F.

3. Turn the heat up to 350°F and cook for 5 to 10 minutes to make the skin crisp.

4. Remove from the smoker, serve immediately and enjoy!

Roasted Tin Foil Dinners

Servings: 4

Cooking Time: 25 Minutes

Ingredients:
- 4 boneless, skinless chicken breast
- Chicken Rub
- 1/2 Pound new potatoes, quartered
- 8 Ounce cremini mushrooms, cleaned and quartered
- salt and pepper
- 1/2 Pound green beans, ends trimmed
- 1 Medium lemon, cut into 3/4 inch slices

Directions:

1. Supply your smoker with wood pellets and follow the start-up procedure. Preheat the grill, with the lid closed, to 400° F.

2. Season chicken breast with salt, pepper and Traeger Chicken Rub. Place the potatoes, mushrooms and chicken in the middle of a large sheet of foil, season with more salt and pepper as needed, and wrap up tightly.

3. Place foil pack directly on the grill grate and cook for 15 minutes. Grill: 400 °F

4. Open up the foil pack and add green beans, lemon and additional salt and pepper, if needed. Wrap back up and return to the Traeger for an additional 10 minutes. Grill: 400 °F

5. Remove from the Traeger, open packet and enjoy!

Sweet And Spicy Smoked Wings

Servings: 2-4

Cooking Time: 85 Minutes

Ingredients:
- 1 pound chicken wings
- 1 batch Sweet and Spicy Cinnamon Rub

➢ 1 cup barbecue sauce

Directions:

1. Supply your smoker with wood pellets and follow the start-up procedure. Preheat the grill, with the lid closed, to 325°F.

2. Season the chicken wings with the rub. Using your hands, work the rub into the meat.

3. Place the wings directly on the grill grate and cook until they reach an internal temperature of 165°F.

4. Transfer the wings into an aluminum pan. Add the barbecue sauce and stir to coat the wings.

5. Reduce the grill's temperature to 250°F and put the pan on the grill. Smoke the wings for 1 hour more, uncovered. Remove the wings from the grill and serve immediately.

Bbq Pulled Turkey Sandwiches

Servings: 6
Cooking Time: 120 Minutes

Ingredients:
➢ 6 Whole Turkey Thighs
➢ Pork & Poultry Rub
➢ 1 1/2 Cup chicken broth
➢ 1 Cup 'Que BBQ Sauce
➢ 6 Whole Kaiser Buns, Split

Directions:

1. Season turkey thighs on both sides with the Traeger Pork & Poultry rub.

2. Supply your smoker with wood pellets and follow the start-up procedure. Preheat the grill, with the lid closed, to 180° F.

3. Arrange the turkey thighs directly on the grill grate and smoke for 30 minutes.

4. Transfer the thighs to a sturdy disposable aluminum foil or roasting pan. Pour the broth around the thighs. Cover the pan with foil or a lid.

5. Increase temperature to 325°F and preheat, lid closed. Roast the thighs until they reach an internal temperature of 180°F. Grill: 325 °F Probe: 180 °F

6. Remove pan from the grill, but leave grill on. Let the turkey thighs cool slightly until they can be comfortably handled.

7. Pour off the drippings and reserve. Remove the skin and discard.

8. Pull the turkey meat into shreds with your fingers and return the meat to the roasting pan.

9. Add 1 cup or more of your favorite Traeger BBQ Sauce along with some of the drippings.

10. Recover the pan with foil and reheat the BBQ turkey on the Traeger for 20 to 30 minutes.

11. Serve with toasted buns if desired. Enjoy!

Bourbon Chicken Waffles

Servings: 8
Cooking Time: 30 Minutes

Ingredients:
➢ 1 Shot Of Bourbon
➢ 3 Cups Bread Crumbs
➢ 4 Horizontally Half Sliced Boneless, Skinless Chicken Breast
➢ Butter Flavored Cooking Spray
➢ 3 Eggs
➢ 1 Tsp Garlic Powder
➢ 1 Tsp Paprika, Powder
➢ Red Velvet Cake Mix
➢ 16 Oz. Reduced Fat Sour Cream
➢ Sweet Rib Rub
➢ ¼ Cup Vegetable Oil
➢ 1 ¼ Cup Water
➢ 1 Tbsp Worcestershire Sauce

Directions:

1. Supply your smoker with wood pellets and follow the start-up procedure. Preheat the grill, with the lid closed, to 350° F. If you're using a gas or charcoal grill, set up the grill for medium heat.

2. In a large bowl, combine the sour cream, bourbon, Worcestershire sauce, paprika, garlic powder, and Sweet Rib Rub seasoning. Add the chicken, turn the chicken breasts to coat, and cover the bowl. Refrigerate for 4-12 hrs.

3. Remove the chicken from the refrigerator and drain the marinade from the chicken. Mix together 3 cups bread crumbs and 2 tbsp Sweet Rib Rub. Mix the coating together and bread the chicken breasts.

4. Moisten a paper towel with cooking oil and using a pair of tongs, lightly grease the grill rack.

5. Grill or smoke until the internal temperature of the chicken reaches 170°F and the chicken is crispy and golden brown.

6. While the chicken is cooking, mix the eggs, vegetable oil, water, and red velvet cake mix in a bowl with the electric mixer.

7. Add the mix into the waffle iron and cook. Make as many waffles as the mix allows.

8. On a plate, place the cooked chicken on top of the waffles and top with maple syrup or honey.

Baked Prosciutto-wrapped Chicken Breast With Spinach And Boursin

Servings: 4

Cooking Time: 60 Minutes

Ingredients:

- 1 Tablespoon olive oil
- 10 Ounce baby spinach leaves, washed and dried
- 2 Whole packs (5.2 oz) Boursin Garlic & Fine Herbs Gournay Cheese
- 2 Pound boneless, skinless chicken breasts
- Pork & Poultry Rub
- 14 Slices prosciutto

Directions:

1. Heat olive oil in a medium sauté pan. Add spinach and sauté until wilted, about 3 to 5 minutes. Transfer to a strainer and squeeze out excess liquid. Place spinach and cheese in a medium bowl. Mix well and set aside.

2. Butterfly each chicken breast and open like a book. Cover with plastic wrap and using a meat mallet, pound out thinly. Season the chicken with Pork & Poultry Rub.

3. Lay a sheet of plastic wrap about 2 feet long down on a flat, clean surface. Lay down slices of prosciutto, slightly overlapping and double-wide. Place the chicken on top of the prosciutto leaving a 1- 1/2 inch border.

4. Spread the spinach mixture on top of the chicken. Roll it up tightly to create a log. Tie off the ends tightly and transfer to the refrigerator. Refrigerate 2 to 3 hours or overnight.

5. Supply your smoker with wood pellets and follow the start-up procedure. Preheat the grill, with the lid closed, to 300° F.

6. Carefully remove the plastic wrap and place directly on the grill grate. Bake for an hour and a half, or until the internal temperature reaches 162°F to 165°F. Remove from Traeger and let rest for 10 minutes before slicing. Enjoy! Grill: 300 ˚F Probe: 162 ˚F

Hot Turkey Sandwich With Gravy

Servings: 4

Cooking Time: 10 Minutes

Ingredients:

- 8 Slices Bread, Sliced
- 1 Cup Gravy, Prepared
- 2 Cups Leftover Turkey, Shredded

Directions:

1. Supply your smoker with wood pellets and follow the start-up procedure. Preheat the grill, with the lid closed, to 400° F.

2. Place the BBQ Grill Mat on the grates of your preheated grill and lay the shredded turkey evenly across the mat to reheat for about 10 minutes.

3. Prepare or reheat the gravy. You"ll want to have the gravy warmed and ready as soon as the turkey is reheated and the bread is toasted.

4. Hold each slice of bread over the flame broiler to toast to your liking.

5. When all of your ingredients are hot, scoop 1/2 cup of the shredded turkey onto a piece of bread, generously cover with gravy and top with another piece of toasted bread. Serve immediately.

Green Chile Chicken Enchiladas

Servings: 6
Cooking Time: 45 Minutes

Ingredients:

- 2 Cups Chicken, Shredded
- 1 (12 Oz) Package Colby Jack Cheese, Shredded
- 1 Enchilada Sauce, Can
- 1 Can Green Chile, Drained
- 1 Onion, Diced
- 1 Tablespoon Sweet Rib Rub
- 1 Cup Sour Cream
- 1 Package Flour Tortilla

Directions:

1. Supply your smoker with wood pellets and follow the start-up procedure. Preheat the grill, with the lid open, to 300° F.

2. In a bowl, mix - the chicken, green chiles, Sweet Heat seasoning, sour cream, diced onion, and half the bag of shredded cheese.

3. Place a large spoonful of the chicken mixture in the center of a tortilla and roll it up. Repeat with the remaining tortillas, then place in the baking pan, and pour the enchilada sauce over the tortilla pans. Top with the remainder of the shredded cheese.

4. Wrap the top of the pan tightly in aluminum foil and grill for 45 minutes or until the enchilada sauce is bubbly. Remove from the grill and serve.

APPETIZERS AND SNACKS

Chicken Wings With Teriyaki Glaze

Servings: 4

Cooking Time: 50 Minutes

Ingredients:

- 16 large chicken wings, about 3lb (1.4kg) total
- 1 to 1½ tbsp toasted sesame oil
- for the glaze
- ½ cup light soy sauce or tamari
- ¼ cup sake or sugar-free dark-colored soda
- ¼ cup light brown sugar or low-carb substitute
- 2 tbsp mirin or 1 tbsp honey
- 1 garlic clove, peeled, minced or grated
- 2 tsp minced fresh ginger
- 1 tsp cornstarch mixed with 1 tbsp distilled water (optional)
- for serving
- 1 tbsp toasted sesame seeds
- 2 scallions, trimmed, white and green parts sliced sharply diagonally

Directions:

1. Supply your smoker with wood pellets and follow the start-up procedure. Preheat the grill, with the lid closed, to 350° F.

2. Place the chicken wings in a large bowl, add the sesame oil, and turn the wings to coat thoroughly.

3. Place the wings on the grate at an angle to the bars. Grill for 20 minutes and then turn. Continue to cook until the wings are nicely browned and the meat is no longer pink at the bone, about 20 minutes more.

4. To make the glaze, in a saucepan on the stovetop over medium-high heat, combine the ingredients and bring the mixture to a boil. Reduce the glaze by 1⁄3, about 6 to 8 minutes. If you prefer your glaze to be glossy and thick, add the cornstarch and water mixture to the glaze and cook until it coats the back of a spoon, about 1 to 2 minutes more.

5. Transfer the wings to an aluminum foil roasting pan. Pour the glaze over them, turning to coat thoroughly. Place the pan on the grate and cook the wings until the glaze sets, about 5 to 10 minutes.

6. Transfer the wings to a platter. Scatter the sesame seeds and scallions over the top. Serve with plenty of napkins.

Bacon-wrapped Jalapeño Poppers

Servings: 12

Cooking Time: 30 Minutes

Ingredients:

- 8 ounces cream cheese, softened
- ½ cup shredded Cheddar cheese
- ¼ cup chopped scallions
- 1 teaspoon chipotle chile powder or regular chili powder
- 1 teaspoon garlic powder
- 1 teaspoon salt
- 18 large jalapeño peppers, stemmed, seeded, and halved lengthwise
- 1 pound bacon (precooked works well)

Directions:

1. Supply your smoker with wood pellets and follow the start-up procedure. Preheat, with the

lid closed, to 350°F. Line a baking sheet with aluminum foil.

2. In a small bowl, combine the cream cheese, Cheddar cheese, scallions, chipotle powder, garlic powder, and salt.

3. Stuff the jalapeño halves with the cheese mixture.

4. Cut the bacon into pieces big enough to wrap around the stuffed pepper halves.

5. Wrap the bacon around the peppers and place on the prepared baking sheet.

6. Put the baking sheet on the grill grate, close the lid, and smoke the peppers for 30 minutes, or until the cheese is melted and the bacon is cooked through and crisp.

7. Let the jalapeño poppers cool for 3 to 5 minutes. Serve warm.

Bacon Pork Pinwheels (kansas Lollipops)

Servings: 4-6

Cooking Time: 20 Minutes

Ingredients:

- ➢ 1 Whole Pork Loin, boneless
- ➢ To Taste salt and pepper
- ➢ To Taste Greek Seasoning
- ➢ 4 Slices bacon
- ➢ To Taste The Ultimate BBQ Sauce

Directions:

1. When ready to cook, start the smoker and set temperature to 500F. Preheat, lid closed, for 10 to 15 minutes.

2. Trim pork loin of any unwanted silver skin or fat. Using a sharp knife, cut pork loin length wise, into 4 long strips.

3. Lay pork flat, then season with salt, pepper and Cavender's Greek Seasoning.

4. Flip the pork strips over and layer bacon on unseasoned side. Begin tightly rolling the pork strips, with bacon being rolled up on the inside.

5. Secure a skewer all the way through each pork roll to secure it in place. Set the pork rolls down on grill and cook for 15 minutes.

6. Brush BBQ Sauce over the pork. Turn each skewer over, then coat the other side. Let pork cook for another 5-10 minutes, depending on thickness of your pork. Enjoy!

Bayou Wings With Cajun Rémoulade

Servings: 8

Cooking Time: 40 Minutes

Ingredients:

- ➢ 16 large whole chicken wings or 32 drumettes and flats, about 3lb (1.4kg) total
- ➢ for the rub
- ➢ 1 tbsp kosher salt
- ➢ 1 tsp freshly ground black pepper
- ➢ 1 tsp paprika
- ➢ ½ tsp ground cayenne, plus more
- ➢ ½ tsp garlic powder
- ➢ ½ tsp celery salt
- ➢ ½ tsp dried thyme
- ➢ 2 tbsp vegetable oil
- ➢ for the rémoulade
- ➢ 1¼ cups reduced-fat mayo
- ➢ ¼ cup Creole-style or whole grain mustard
- ➢ 2 tbsp horseradish
- ➢ 2 tbsp pickle relish
- ➢ 1 tbsp freshly squeezed lemon juice
- ➢ 1 tsp paprika, plus more
- ➢ 1 tsp hot sauce, plus more
- ➢ 1 tsp Worcestershire sauce
- ➢ coarse salt

- ➢ for serving
- ➢ lemon wedges
- ➢ pickled okra (optional)

Directions:

1. Supply your smoker with wood pellets and follow the start-up procedure. Preheat the grill, with the lid closed, to 350° F.

2. If using whole wings, cut through the two joints, separating them into drumettes, flats, and wing tips. (Discard the wing tips or save them for chicken stock.) Alternatively, leave the wings whole. Place the chicken in a resealable plastic bag.

3. In a small bowl, make the rub by combining the ingredients. Mix well. Pour the rub over the wings and toss them to thoroughly coat. Refrigerate for 2 hours.

4. In a small bowl, make the Cajun rémoulade by whisking together the mayo, mustard, horseradish, pickle relish, lemon juice, paprika, hot sauce, and Worcestershire. Season with salt to taste. The mixture should be highly seasoned. Transfer to a serving bowl and lightly dust with paprika. Cover and refrigerate until ready to serve.

5. Remove the wings from the refrigerator and allow the excess marinade to drip off. Place the wings on the grate at an angle to the bars. Grill for 20 minutes and then turn. (They'll brown more evenly but will also have less of a tendency to stick.) Continue to cook until the wings are nicely browned and the meat is no longer pink at the bone, about 20 minutes more.

6. Remove the wings from the grill and pile them on a platter. Serve with the Cajun rémoulade, lemon wedges, and pickled okra (if using).

Pulled Pork Loaded Nachos

Servings: 4

Cooking Time: 10 Minutes

Ingredients:

- ➢ 2 cups leftover smoked pulled pork
- ➢ 1 small sweet onion, diced
- ➢ 1 medium tomato, diced
- ➢ 1 jalapeño pepper, seeded and diced
- ➢ 1 garlic clove, minced
- ➢ 1 teaspoon salt
- ➢ 1 teaspoon freshly ground black pepper
- ➢ 1 bag tortilla chips
- ➢ 1 cup shredded Cheddar cheese
- ➢ ½ cup The Ultimate BBQ Sauce, divided
- ➢ ½ cup shredded jalapeño Monterey Jack cheese
- ➢ Juice of ½ lime
- ➢ 1 avocado, halved, pitted, and sliced
- ➢ 2 tablespoons sour cream
- ➢ 1 tablespoon chopped fresh cilantro

Directions:

1. Supply your smoker with wood pellets and follow the start-up procedure. Preheat, with the lid closed, to 375°F.

2. Heat the pulled pork in the microwave.

3. In a medium bowl, combine the onion, tomato, jalapeño, garlic, salt, and pepper, and set aside.

4. Arrange half of the tortilla chips in a large cast iron skillet. Spread half of the warmed pork on top and cover with the Cheddar cheese. Top with half of the onion-jalapeño mixture, then drizzle with ¼ cup of barbecue sauce.

5. Layer on the remaining tortilla chips, then the remaining pork and the Monterey Jack cheese. Top with the remaining onion-jalapeño mixture

and drizzle with the remaining ¼ cup of barbecue sauce.

6. Place the skillet on the grill, close the lid, and smoke for about 10 minutes, or until the cheese is melted and bubbly. (Watch to make sure your chips don't burn!)

7. Squeeze the lime juice over the nachos, top with the avocado slices and sour cream, and garnish with the cilantro before serving hot.

Citrus-infused Marinated Olives

Servings: 6

Cooking Time: 30 Minutes

Ingredients:

➢ 1½ cups mixed brined olives, with pits

➢ ½ cup extra virgin olive oil

➢ 1 tbsp freshly squeezed lemon juice

➢ 1 garlic clove, peeled and thinly sliced

➢ 1 tsp smoked Spanish paprika

➢ 2 sprigs of fresh rosemary

➢ 2 sprigs of fresh thyme

➢ 2 bay leaves, fresh or dried

➢ 1 small dried red chili pepper, deseeded and flesh crumbled, or ¼ tsp crushed red pepper flakes

➢ 3 strips of orange zest

➢ 3 strips of lemon zest

Directions:

1. Supply your smoker with wood pellets and follow the start-up procedure. Preheat the grill, with the lid closed, to 180° F.

2. Drain the olives, reserving 1 tablespoon of brine. Spread the olives in a single layer in an aluminum foil roasting pan. Place the pan on the grate and cook the olives for 30 minutes, stirring the olives or shaking the pan once or twice.

3. In a small saucepan on the stovetop over low heat, warm the olive oil. Whisk in the lemon juice and the reserved 1 tablespoon of brine. Stir in the garlic and paprika. Add the rosemary, thyme, bay leaves, chili pepper, and orange and lemon zests. Warm over low heat for 10 minutes. Remove the saucepan from the heat.

4. Transfer the olives and olive oil mixture to a pint jar. Tuck the aromatics around the sides of the jar. Let cool and then cover and refrigerate for up to 5 days. Let the olives come to room temperature before serving.

Chorizo Queso Fundido

Servings: 4-6

Cooking Time: 20 Minutes

Ingredients:

➢ 1 poblano chile

➢ 1 cup chopped queso quesadilla or queso Oaxaca

➢ 1 cup shredded Monterey Jack cheese

➢ ¼ cup milk

➢ 1 tablespoon all-purpose flour

➢ 2 (4-ounce) links Mexican chorizo sausage, casings removed

➢ ⅓ cup beer

➢ 1 tablespoon unsalted butter

➢ 1 small red onion, chopped

➢ ½ cup whole kernel corn

➢ 2 serrano chiles or jalapeño peppers, stemmed, seeded, and coarsely chopped

➢ 1 tablespoon minced garlic

➢ 1 tablespoon freshly squeezed lime juice

➢ 1 teaspoon ground cumin

➢ 1 teaspoon salt

➢ 1 teaspoon freshly ground black pepper

➢ 1 tablespoon chopped fresh cilantro

- ➢ 1 tablespoon chopped scallions
- ➢ Tortilla chips, for serving

Directions:

1. Supply your smoker with wood pellets and follow the start-up procedure. Preheat, with the lid closed, to 350°F.

2. On the smoker or over medium-high heat on the stove top, place the poblano directly on the grate (or burner) to char for 1 to 2 minutes, turning as needed. Remove from heat and place in a closed-up lunch-size paper bag for 2 minutes to sweat and further loosen the skin.

3. Remove the skin and coarsely chop the poblano, removing the seeds; set aside.

4. In a bowl, combine the queso quesadilla, Monterey Jack, milk, and flour; set aside.

5. On the stove top, in a cast iron skillet over medium heat, cook and crumble the chorizo for about 2 minutes.

6. Transfer the cooked chorizo to a small, grill-safe pan and place over indirect heat on the smoker.

7. Place the cast iron skillet on the preheated grill grate. Pour in the beer and simmer for a few minutes, loosening and stirring in any remaining sausage bits from the pan.

8. Add the butter to the pan, then add the cheese mixture a little at a time, stirring constantly.

9. When the cheese is smooth, stir in the onion, corn, serrano chiles, garlic, lime juice, cuvmin, salt, and pepper. Stir in the reserved chopped charred poblano.

10. Close the lid and smoke for 15 to 20 minutes to infuse the queso with smoke flavor and further cook the vegetables.

11. When the cheese is bubbly, top with the chorizo mixture and garnish with the cilantro and scallions.

12. Serve the chorizo queso fundido hot with tortilla chips.

Grilled Guacamole

Servings: 6
Cooking Time: 30 Minutes

Ingredients:
- ➢ 3 large avocados, halved and pitted
- ➢ 1 lime, halved
- ➢ ½ jalapeño, deseeded and deveined
- ➢ ½ small white or red onion, peeled
- ➢ 2 garlic cloves, peeled and skewered on a toothpick
- ➢ 1 tsp coarse salt, plus more
- ➢ 1½ tbsp reduced-fat mayo
- ➢ 2 tbsp chopped fresh cilantro
- ➢ 2 tbsp crumbled queso fresco (optional)
- ➢ tortilla chips

Directions:

1. Supply your smoker with wood pellets and follow the start-up procedure. Preheat the grill, with the lid closed, to 225° F.

2. Place the avocados, lime, jalapeño, and onion cut sides down on the grate. Use the toothpicks to balance the garlic cloves between the bars. Smoke for 30 minutes. (You want the vegetables to retain most of their rawness.)

3. Transfer everything to a cutting board. Remove the garlic cloves from the toothpick and roughly chop. Sprinkle with the salt and continue to mince the garlic until it begins to form a paste. Scrape the garlic and salt into a large bowl.

4. Scoop the avocado flesh from the peels into the bowl. Squeeze the juice of ½ lime over the

avocado. Mash the avocados but leave them somewhat chunky. Finely dice the jalapeño. Dice 2 tablespoons of onion. (Reserve the remaining onion for another use.) Add the jalapeño, onion, mayo, and cilantro to the bowl. Stir gently to combine. Taste for seasoning, adding more salt, lime juice, and jalapeño as desired.

5. Transfer the guacamole to a serving bowl. Top with the queso fresco (if using). Serve with tortilla chips.

Pigs In A Blanket

Servings: 4-6
Cooking Time: 15 Minutes

Ingredients:

- 2 Tablespoon Poppy Seeds
- 1 Tablespoon Dried Minced Onion
- 2 Teaspoon garlic, minced
- 2 Tablespoon Sesame Seeds
- 1 Teaspoon salt
- 8 Ounce Original Crescent Dough
- 1/4 Cup Dijon mustard
- 1 Large egg, beaten

Directions:

1. When ready to cook, start your smoker at 350 degrees F, and preheat with lid closed, 10 to 15 minutes.

2. Mix together poppy seeds, dried minced onion, dried minced garlic, salt and sesame seeds. Set aside.

3. Cut each triangle of crescent roll dough into thirds lengthwise, making 3 small strips from each roll.

4. Brush the dough strips lightly with Dijon mustard. Put the mini hot dogs on 1 end of the dough and roll up.

5. Arrange them, seam side down, on a greased baking pan. Brush with egg wash and sprinkle with seasoning mixture.

6. Bake in smoker until golden brown, about 12 to 15 minutes.

7. Serve with mustard or dipping sauce of your choice. Enjoy!

Simple Cream Cheese Sausage Balls

Servings: 5
Cooking Time: 30 Minutes

Ingredients:

- 1 pound ground hot sausage, uncooked
- 8 ounces cream cheese, softened
- 1 package mini filo dough shells

Directions:

1. Supply your smoker with wood pellets and follow the start-up procedure. Preheat, with the lid closed, to 350°F.

2. In a large bowl, using your hands, thoroughly mix together the sausage and cream cheese until well blended.

3. Place the filo dough shells on a rimmed perforated pizza pan or into a mini muffin tin.

4. Roll the sausage and cheese mixture into 1-inch balls and place into the filo shells.

5. Place the pizza pan or mini muffin tin on the grill, close the lid, and smoke the sausage balls for 30 minutes, or until cooked through and the sausage is no longer pink.

6. Plate and serve warm.

Deviled Eggs With Smoked Paprika

Servings: 6
Cooking Time: 30 Minutes

Ingredients:

- 6 large eggs
- 3 tbsp reduced-fat mayo, plus more
- 1 tsp Dijon or yellow mustard
- ½ tsp Spanish smoked paprika or regular paprika, plus more
- dash of hot sauce
- coarse salt
- freshly ground black pepper
- for garnishing
- small sprigs of fresh parsley, dill, tarragon, or cilantro
- chopped chives
- minced scallions
- Mustard Caviar
- sliced green or black olives
- celery leaves
- sliced radishes
- diced bell peppers
- sliced cherry tomatoes
- fresh or pickled jalapeños
- sliced or diced pickles
- slivers of sun-dried tomatoes
- bacon crumbles
- smoked salmon
- Hawaiian black salt
- Caviar

Directions:

1. Supply your smoker with wood pellets and follow the start-up procedure. Preheat the grill, with the lid closed, to 180° F.

2. On the stovetop over medium-high heat, bring a saucepan of water to a boil. (Make sure there's enough water in the saucepan to cover the eggs by 1 inch [5cm].) Use a slotted spoon to gently lower the eggs into the water. Lower the heat to maintain a simmer. Set a timer for 13 minutes.

3. Prepare an ice bath by combining ice and cold water in a large bowl. Carefully transfer the eggs to the ice bath when the timer goes off.

4. When the eggs are cool enough to handle, gently tap them all over to crack the shell. Carefully peel the eggs. Rinse under cold running water to remove any clinging bits of shell, but don't dry the eggs. (A damp surface will help the smoke adhere to the egg whites.)

5. Place the eggs on the grate and smoke until the eggs take on a light brown patina from the smoke, about 25 minutes. Transfer the eggs to a cutting board, handling them as little as possible.

6. Slice each egg in half lengthwise with a sharp knife. Wipe any yolk off the blade before slicing the next egg. Gently remove the yolks and place them in a food processor. Pulse to break up the yolks. Add the mayo, mustard, paprika, and hot sauce. Season with salt and pepper to taste. Pulse until the filling is smooth. Add additional mayo 1 teaspoon at a time if the mixture is a little dry. (It shouldn't be too loose either.)

7. Spoon the filling into each egg half or pipe it in using a small resealable plastic bag. You can also use a pastry bag fitted with a fluted tip.

8. Place the eggs on a platter and lightly dust with paprika. Accompany with one or more of the suggested garnishes.

Smoked Cashews

Servings: 6
Cooking Time: 60 Minutes

Ingredients:

➢ 1 pound roasted, salted cashews

Directions:

1. Supply your smoker with wood pellets and follow the start-up procedure. Preheat the grill, with the lid closed, to 120°F.

2. Pour the cashews onto a rimmed baking sheet and smoke for 1 hour, stirring once about halfway through the smoking time.

3. Remove the cashews from the grill, let cool, and store in an airtight container for as long as you can resist.

Pig Pops (sweet-hot Bacon On A Stick)

Servings: 24
Cooking Time: 30 Minutes

Ingredients:

➢ Nonstick cooking spray, oil, or butter, for greasing
➢ 2 pounds thick-cut bacon (24 slices)
➢ 24 metal skewers
➢ 1 cup packed light brown sugar
➢ 2 to 3 teaspoons cayenne pepper
➢ ½ cup maple syrup, divided

Directions:

1. Supply your smoker with wood pellets and follow the start-up procedure. Preheat, with the lid closed, to 350°F.

2. Coat a disposable aluminum foil baking sheet with cooking spray, oil, or butter.

3. Thread each bacon slice onto a metal skewer and place on the prepared baking sheet.

4. In a medium bowl, stir together the brown sugar and cayenne.

5. Baste the top sides of the bacon with ¼ cup of maple syrup.

6. Sprinkle half of the brown sugar mixture over the bacon.

7. Place the baking sheet on the grill, close the lid, and smoke for 15 to 30 minutes.

8. Using tongs, flip the bacon skewers. Baste with the remaining ¼ cup of maple syrup and top with the remaining brown sugar mixture.

9. Continue smoking with the lid closed for 10 to 15 minutes, or until crispy. You can eyeball the bacon and smoke to your desired doneness, but the actual ideal internal temperature for bacon is 155°F

10. Using tongs, carefully remove the bacon skewers from the grill. Let cool completely before handling.

Chuckwagon Beef Jerky

Servings: 6
Cooking Time: 300 Minutes

Ingredients:

➢ 2½lb (1.2kg) boneless top or bottom round steak, sirloin tip, flank steak, or venison
➢ 1 cup sugar-free dark-colored soda
➢ 1 cup cold brewed coffee
➢ ½ cup light soy sauce
➢ ¼ cup Worcestershire sauce
➢ 2 tbsp whiskey (optional)
➢ 2 tsp chili powder
➢ 1½ tsp garlic salt
➢ 1 tsp onion powder
➢ 1 tsp pink curing salt

Directions:

1. Slice the meat into ¼-inch-thick (.5cm) strips, trimming off any visible fat or gristle. (Slice against the grain for more tender jerky and with the grain for chewier jerky.) Place the meat in a large resealable plastic bag.

2. In a small bowl, whisk together the soda, coffee, soy sauce, Worcestershire sauce, whiskey (if using), chili powder, garlic salt, onion powder, and curing salt (if using). Whisk until the salt dissolves. Pour the mixture over the meat and reseal the bag. Refrigerate for 24 to 48 hours, turning the bag several times to redistribute the brine.

3. Supply your smoker with wood pellets and follow the start-up procedure. Preheat the grill, with the lid closed, to 150° F.

4. Drain the meat and discard the brine. Place the strips of meat in a single layer on paper towels and blot any excess moisture.

5. Place the meat in a single layer on the grate and smoke for 4 to 5 hours, turning once or twice. (If you're aware of hot spots on your grate, rotate the strips so they smoke evenly.) To test for doneness, bend one or two pieces in the middle. They should be dry but still somewhat pliant. Or simply eat a piece to see if it's done to your liking.

6. For the best texture, when you remove the meat from the grill, place the still-warm jerky in a resealable plastic bag and let rest for 30 minutes. (You might see condensation form on the inside of the bag, but the moisture will be reabsorbed by the meat.) Or let the meat cool completely and then store in a resealable plastic bag or covered container. The jerky will last a few days at room temperature but will last longer (up to 2 weeks) if refrigerated.

Smoked Cheese

Servings: 4
Cooking Time: 150 Minutes

Ingredients:

➢ 1 (2-pound) block medium Cheddar cheese, or your favorite cheese, quartered lengthwise

Directions:

1. Supply your smoker with wood pellets and follow the start-up procedure. Preheat the grill, with the lid closed, to 90°F.

2. Place the cheese directly on the grill grate and smoke for 2 hours, 30 minutes, checking frequently to be sure it's not melting. If the cheese begins to melt, try flipping it. If that doesn't help, remove it from the grill and refrigerate for about 1 hour and then return it to the cold smoker.

3. Remove the cheese, place it in a zip-top bag, and refrigerate overnight.

4. Slice the cheese and serve with crackers, or grate it and use for making a smoked mac and cheese.

Roasted Red Pepper Dip

Servings: 8
Cooking Time: 45 Minutes

Ingredients:

➢ 4 red bell peppers, halved, destemmed, and deseeded
➢ 1 cup English walnuts, divided
➢ 1 small white onion, peeled and coarsely chopped
➢ 2 garlic cloves, peeled and smashed with a chef's knife
➢ ¼ cup extra virgin olive oil, plus more
➢ 1 tbsp balsamic vinegar or balsamic glaze
➢ 1 tsp honey (eliminate if using balsamic glaze)

- ➢ 1 tsp coarse salt, plus more
- ➢ 1 tsp ground cumin
- ➢ 1 tsp smoked paprika
- ➢ ½ to 1 tsp Aleppo red pepper flakes, plus more
- ➢ ¼ cup fresh white breadcrumbs (optional)
- ➢ distilled water (optional)
- ➢ assorted crudités or wedges of pita bread

Directions:

1. Supply your smoker with wood pellets and follow the start-up procedure. Preheat the grill, with the lid closed, to 400° F.

2. Place the peppers skin side down on the grate and grill until the skins blister and the flesh softens, about 30 minutes. Transfer the peppers to a bowl and cover with plastic wrap. Let cool to room temperature. Remove the skins with a paring knife or your fingers. Coarsely chop or tear the peppers.

3. Place ¾ cup of walnuts in an aluminum foil roasting pan. Place the pan on the grate and toast for 10 to 15 minutes, stirring twice. Remove the pan from the grill and let the walnuts cool.

4. Place the peppers, onion, garlic, and walnuts in a food processor fitted with the chopping blade. Pulse several times. Add the olive oil, balsamic vinegar, honey, salt, cumin, paprika, and red pepper flakes. Process until the mixture is fairly smooth. Taste for seasoning, adding more salt or red pepper flakes (if desired). (If the mixture is too loose, add breadcrumbs until the texture is to your liking. If it's too thick, add olive oil or water 1 tablespoon at a time.)

5. Transfer the dip to a serving bowl. Use the back of a spoon to make a shallow depression in the center. Top with the remaining ¼ cup of walnuts and drizzle olive oil in the depression. Serve with crudités or pita bread.

Delicious Deviled Crab Appetizer

Servings: 30

Cooking Time: 10 Minutes

Ingredients:

- ➢ Nonstick cooking spray, oil, or butter, for greasing
- ➢ 1 cup panko breadcrumbs, divided
- ➢ 1 cup canned corn, drained
- ➢ ½ cup chopped scallions, divided
- ➢ ½ red bell pepper, finely chopped
- ➢ 16 ounces jumbo lump crabmeat
- ➢ ¾ cup mayonnaise, divided
- ➢ 1 egg, beaten
- ➢ 1 teaspoon salt
- ➢ 1 teaspoon freshly ground black pepper
- ➢ 2 teaspoons cayenne pepper, divided
- ➢ Juice of 1 lemon

Directions:

1. Supply your smoker with wood pellets and follow the start-up procedure. Preheat, with the lid closed, to 425°F.

2. Spray three 12-cup mini muffin pans with cooking spray and divide ½ cup of the panko between 30 of the muffin cups, pressing into the bottoms and up the sides. (Work in batches, if necessary, depending on the number of pans you have.)

3. In a medium bowl, combine the corn, ¼ cup of scallions, the bell pepper, crabmeat, half of the mayonnaise, the egg, salt, pepper, and 1 teaspoon of cayenne pepper.

4. Gently fold in the remaining ½ cup of breadcrumbs and divide the mixture between the prepared mini muffin cups.

5. Place the pans on the grill grate, close the lid, and smoke for 10 minutes, or until golden brown.

6. In a small bowl, combine the lemon juice and the remaining mayonnaise, scallions, and cayenne pepper to make a sauce.

7. Brush the tops of the mini crab cakes with the sauce and serve hot.

Smoked Turkey Sandwich

Servings: 1
Cooking Time: 15 Minutes

Ingredients:

- 2 slices sourdough bread
- 2 tablespoons butter, at room temperature
- 2 (1-ounce) slices Swiss cheese
- 4 ounces leftover Smoked Turkey
- 1 teaspoon garlic salt

Directions:

1. Supply your smoker with wood pellets and follow the start-up procedure. Preheat the grill, with the lid closed, to 375°F.

2. Coat one side of each bread slice with 1 tablespoon of butter and sprinkle the buttered sides with garlic salt.

3. Place 1 slice of cheese on each unbuttered side of the bread, and then put the turkey on the cheese.

4. Close the sandwich, buttered sides out, and place it directly on the grill grate. Cook for 5 minutes. Flip the sandwich and cook for 5 minutes more. Remove the sandwich from the grill, cut it in half, and serve.

Sriracha & Maple Cashews

Servings: 10
Cooking Time: 60 Minutes

Ingredients:

- 2 tbsp unsalted butter
- 3 tbsp pure maple syrup
- 1 tbsp sriracha
- 1 tsp coarse salt (use only if nuts are unsalted)
- 2½ cups unsalted cashews

Directions:

1. Supply your smoker with wood pellets and follow the start-up procedure. Preheat the grill, with the lid closed, to 250° F.

2. In a small saucepan on the stovetop over low heat, melt the butter. Add the maple syrup, sriracha, and salt (if using). Stir until combined. Add the nuts and stir gently to coat thoroughly.

3. Spread the nuts in a single layer in an aluminum foil roasting pan coated with cooking spray. Place the pan on the grate and smoke the nuts until they're lightly toasted, about 1 hour, stirring once or twice.

4. Remove the pan from the grill and let the nuts cool for 15 minutes. They'll be sticky at first but will crisp up. Break them up with your fingers and store at room temperature in an airtight container, such as a lidded glass jar.

Jalapeño Poppers With Chipotle Sour Cream

Servings: 8
Cooking Time: 45 Minutes

Ingredients:

- 3 strips of thin-sliced bacon
- 12 large jalapeños, red, green, or a mix
- 8oz (225g) light cream cheese, at room temperature
- 1 cup shredded pepper Jack, Monterey Jack, or Cheddar cheese
- 1 tsp chili powder
- ½ tsp garlic salt

- ➢ smoked paprika
- ➢ for the sour cream
- ➢ 1¼ cups light sour cream
- ➢ juice of ½ lime
- ➢ ½ to 1 canned chipotle peppers in adobo sauce, finely minced, plus 1 tsp of sauce, plus more
- ➢ 1 tbsp minced fresh cilantro leaves
- ➢ ½ tsp coarse salt, plus more

Directions:

1. Supply your smoker with wood pellets and follow the start-up procedure. Preheat the grill, with the lid closed, to 375° F.

2. Line a rimmed sheet pan with aluminum foil and place a wire rack on top. Place the bacon in a single layer on the wire rack. Place the pan on the grate and grill until the bacon is crisp and golden brown, about 20 minutes. Transfer the bacon to paper towels to cool and then crumble. Set aside.

3. In a small bowl, make the chipotle sour cream by whisking together the ingredients. Add more salt, chipotle peppers, or adobe sauce to taste. Cover and refrigerate.

4. Slice the jalapeños lengthwise through their stems. Scrape out the veins and seeds with the edge of a small metal spoon.

5. In a small bowl, beat together the cream cheese, shredded cheese, chili powder, and garlic salt. Stir in the crumbled bacon. Mound the cream cheese mixture in the jalapeño halves. Line another rimmed sheet pan with aluminum foil and place a wire rack on top. Place the jalapeños filled side up in a single layer on the wire rack.

6. Place the sheet pan on the grate and roast the jalapeños until the filling has melted and the peppers have softened, about 20 to 25 minutes. (They should no longer look bright in color.)

Remove the pan from the grill and let the peppers rest for 5 minutes.

7. Transfer the poppers to a platter and lightly dust with paprika. Serve with the chipotle sour cream.

Cold-smoked Cheese

Servings: 6
Cooking Time: 180 Minutes

Ingredients:

- ➢ 2lb (1kg) well-chilled hard or semi-hard cheese, such as:
- ➢ Edam
- ➢ Gouda
- ➢ Cheddar
- ➢ Monterey Jack
- ➢ pepper Jack
- ➢ goat cheese
- ➢ fresh mozzarella
- ➢ Muenster
- ➢ aged Parmigiano-Reggiano
- ➢ Gruyère
- ➢ blue cheese

Directions:

1. Unwrap the cheese and remove any protective wax or coating. Cut into 4-ounce (110g) portions to increase the surface area.

2. If possible, move your smoker to a shady area. Place 1 resealable plastic bag filled with ice on top of the drip pan. This is especially important on a warm day because you want to keep the interior temperature of the grill between 70 and 90°F (21 and 32°C) or below.

3. Place a grill mat on one side of the grate. Place the cheese on the mat and allow space between each piece.

4. Fill your smoking tube or pellet maze (see Cast Iron Skillets and Grill Pans) with pellets or sawdust and light according to the manufacturer's instructions. Place the smoking tube on the grate near—but not on—the grill mat. When the tube is smoking consistently, close the grill lid.

5. Smoke the cheese for 1 to 3 hours, replacing the pellets or sawdust and ice if necessary. Monitor the temperature and make sure the cheese isn't beginning to melt. Carefully lift the mat with the cheese to a rimmed baking sheet and let the cheese cool completely before handling.

6. Package the smoked cheese in cheese storage paper or bags or vacuum-seal the cheese, labeling each. (While you can wrap the cheese tightly in plastic wrap, the cheese will spoil faster.) Let the cheese rest for at least 2 to 3 days before eating. It will be even better after 2 weeks.

BEEF LAMB AND GAME RECIPES

Smoked Burgers

Servings: 8
Cooking Time: 120 Minutes

Ingredients:

- 2 Pound ground beef
- 1 Tablespoon Worcestershire sauce
- 2 Tablespoon Beef Rub

Directions:

1. Mix ground beef with Worcestershire sauce and Traeger Beef rub.
2. Form beef mixture into 8 hamburger patties.
3. Supply your smoker with wood pellets and follow the start-up procedure. Preheat the grill, with the lid closed, to 180° F.
4. Place patties directly on the grill grate and smoke for 2 hours. Grill: 180 ˚F
5. After 2 hours, remove from grill and serve with your favorite toppings. Enjoy!

Grilled Loco Moco Burger

Servings: 4
Cooking Time: 10 Minutes

Ingredients:

- Ounce ground beef, 80% lean
- 3 Tablespoon kosher salt
- 2 Tablespoon black pepper
- Cup Beef Gravy
- 2 Cup Rice, Cooked
- 4 eggs
- burger buns
- 2 Cup Hawaiian Pasta Salad

Directions:

1. Supply your smoker with wood pellets and follow the start-up procedure. Preheat the grill, with the lid closed, to 375° F.
2. Divide the ground beef into four, 6 oz portions and shape into patties. Season the patties with salt and pepper.
3. Place the patties on the grill and flip after six minutes cook time.
4. Check the internal temperature of the patties. Burgers are done when they reach an internal temperature of 165˚F . Probe: 165 ˚F
5. While the patties are cooking, heat the gravy and the rice. Cook the eggs over easy.
6. To assemble the burger: Start with the bottom of the bun, 1/4 cup rice, 1/4 cup pasta salad, a hamburger patty, gravy, a fried egg, and the top of the bun.
7. Serve while hot. Enjoy!

Texas Smoked Brisket

Servings: 12-15
Cooking Time: 960 Minutes

Ingredients:

- 1 (12-pound) full packer brisket
- 2 tablespoons yellow mustard
- 1 batch Espresso Brisket Rub
- Worcestershire Mop and Spritz, for spritzing

Directions:

1. Supply your smoker with wood pellets and follow the start-up procedure. Preheat the grill, with the lid closed, to 225°F.
2. Using a boning knife, carefully remove all but about ½ inch of the large layer of fat covering one side of your brisket.

3. Coat the brisket all over with mustard and season it with the rub. Using your hands, work the rub into the meat. Pour the mop into a spray bottle.

4. Place the brisket directly on the grill grate and smoke until its internal temperature reaches 195°F, spritzing it every hour with the mop.

5. Pull the brisket from the grill and wrap it completely in aluminum foil or butcher paper. Place the wrapped brisket in a cooler, cover the cooler, and let it rest for 1 or 2 hours.

6. Remove the brisket from the cooler and unwrap it.

7. Separate the brisket point from the flat by cutting along the fat layer and slice the flat. The point can be saved for burnt ends (see Sweet Heat Burnt Ends), or sliced and served as well.

Beef Tenderloin With Tomato Vinaigrette

Servings: 6
Cooking Time: 40 Minutes

Ingredients:

- 1 Whole (1-1/4 to 1-1/2 inch thick) beef tenderloin steaks
- 1 Bottle Prime Rib Rub
- 2/3 Cup extra-virgin olive oil
- salt and pepper
- 1 Teaspoon fresh thyme
- 6 Whole plum tomatoes
- 1 Teaspoon Thyme, minced
- 2 Tablespoon balsamic vinegar

Directions:

1. Supply your smoker with wood pellets and follow the start-up procedure. Preheat the grill, with the lid closed, to 450° F.

2. Tuck the thin end of the tenderloin underneath the roast and secure it with butcher's string. Rub the meat with olive oil and season it with the Prime Rib Rub or salt and pepper. Place the meat on a rack in a shallow roasting pan.

3. Roast in the preheated Traeger for 20 minutes. Adjust the heat to 350F. Roast 20 minutes longer, or to desired degree of doneness (130F for rare; 145F for medium; 155F or higher for well-done). Grill: 350 °F

4. Let rest for 5 minutes before slicing thinly. (If serving cold, thoroughly chill the tenderloin before slicing.) Garnish with sprigs of thyme.

5. To make the vinaigrette, combine the tomatoes, olive oil, balsamic vinegar, and thyme leaves in a blender jar or food processor; puree until smooth. Season to taste with Traeger Prime Rib Rub or salt and pepper.

6. Transfer to a gravy boat and serve with the tenderloin. (Best served the day it's made.)

Smoked Bacon Brisket Flat

Servings: 4
Cooking Time: 480 Minutes

Ingredients:

- 1/2 lbs bacon
- 4 lbs brisket flat, trimmed
- tt lonestar brisket rub

Directions:

1. Supply your smoker with wood pellets and follow the start-up procedure. Preheat the grill, with the lid open, to 250° F. If using a gas or charcoal grill, set it up for low, indirect heat.

2. Place the brisket in a foil-lined aluminum pan. Season the fat side of the brisket with Lonestar Brisket Rub, then flip and season the meat side with additional rub.

3. Transfer the brisket to the grill and smoke for 1 hour.

4. Use tongs to flip the brisket over, so the fat side is up, then drape half the bacon slices over the brisket. Smoke for 2 hours, then remove the browned bacon, and set aside.

5. Lay the remaining raw bacon strips over the brisket, and continue cooking until these new bacon strips are browned and the internal temperature of the brisket reads 202°F, which will likely take an additional 3 to 4 hours cook time.

6. Remove the brisket from the grill, and rest for 1 hour, then slice thin. Serve warm.

Reverse Grilled Potato Bacon Wrapped Steaks

Servings: 2
Cooking Time: 60 Minutes

Ingredients:
➢ 1 Bunch Asparagus
➢ 4 Bacon, Strip
➢ BBQ Sauce
➢ 2 Tbsp Olive Oil
➢ 1 Bag Potato, Baby
➢ 2 - 1" Thick Steak, Bone-In Ribeye

Directions:
1. Supply your smoker with wood pellets and follow the start-up procedure. Preheat the grill, with the lid open, to 250° F.

2. Wrap two pieces of bacon around each steak. Place on the grates of your preheated Grill. You'll want to cook the steaks until the internal temperature reaches 130°F (for medium-rare). Follow these internal temperatures if you'd like to cook your steak more/less done:

3. Rare: 125°F

4. Medium Rare: 130°F

5. Medium: 140°F

6. Well Done: 160°F

7. If you're cooking your steaks medium rare, it will take around 45 minutes. Put your baby potatoes in a cast iron pan, drizzle with oil and place on grill with the steaks. When your steaks reach the desired internal temperature, remove steaks from the grill and let them rest for 15 minutes. In the meantime, open up your Flame Broiler Plate and crank up the grill to HIGH, keeping your potatoes on the grill. Add the asparagus to the top of the potatoes and cook. When the grill is preheated to HIGH, sear each side of the steak for about 1 minute each. Serve immediately with or without BBQ Sauce.

Sweet And Spicy Beef Sirloin Tip Roast

Servings: 8
Cooking Time: 120 Minutes

Ingredients:
➢ 3 Pound beef sirloin tip roast
➢ 2 Tablespoon Beef Rub
➢ 1/2 Cup 'Que BBQ Sauce
➢ 1/4 Cup chili sauce

Directions:
1. Season sirloin tip roast evenly with Traeger Beef Rub on all sides. Let roast rest at room temperature for 30 minutes.

2. Supply your smoker with wood pellets and follow the start-up procedure. Preheat the grill, with the lid closed, to 275° F.

3. Place the roast on the Traeger and cook for about 75 minutes or until the internal temperature reaches 130°F. Grill: 275 °F Probe: 130 °F

4. In a small bowl, combine Traeger 'Que and chili sauce. Once meat has reached 130°F, brush the roast with 1/4 cup of the bbq chili sauce.

5. Continue cooking until internal temperature reaches 140°F. Grill: 275 °F Probe: 140 °F

6. Remove from the grill and place on a cutting board then tent with foil. Let stand 10 minutes or until internal temperature reaches 145°F.

7. Slice roast across the grain into thin slices and brush each slice with remaining sauce. Serve, enjoy!

Venison Bbq Burger By Nikki Boxler

Servings: 4
Cooking Time: 12 Minutes

Ingredients:

➤ 5 Slices bacon
➤ 1 Pound Venison, ground
➤ 1/2 Cup 'Que BBQ Sauce
➤ 1/2 Cup shredded cheddar cheese

Directions:

1. Supply your smoker with wood pellets and follow the start-up procedure. Preheat the grill, with the lid closed, to 350° F.

2. Place bacon slices directly on the grill grate and cook 15 minutes until fat is rendered and bacon is crispy. Remove from grill and let cool. When bacon is cool, break it into pieces.

3. Combine the venison, barbecue sauce, bacon and cheese into a large bowl. Then mix carefully so that the ingredients are spread evenly.

4. Once mixed, press the ground venison into burger patties.

5. Place patties directly on the grill grate and cook until the internal temperature reaches 165 degrees F, flipping halfway through.

6. Once the burgers are done, pair it with your favorite bun and top with your choice of toppings. I personally don't add a bun or condiments as the burger is so good, you don't need them. Enjoy!

Braised Onion Chuck Roast Beef Sandwiches

Servings: 4
Cooking Time: 540 Minutes

Ingredients:

➤ 3 cups beef stock, divided
➤ 2 lbs chuck roast
➤ 4 hoagie rolls, sliced lengthwise
➤ to taste, lone star brisket rub
➤ 1 yellow onion

Directions:

1. Place chuck roast in a glass baking dish. Season with Lone Star Brisket Rub, then cover with plastic wrap and refrigerate overnight.

2. The next day, remove chuck roast from the refrigerator. Supply your smoker with wood pellets and follow the start-up procedure. Preheat the grill, with the lid closed, to 225° F. If using a gas or charcoal grill, set it up for low, indirect heat.

3. Place chuck roast directly on the grill grate, then close the lid and smoke for 3 hours, spraying with 1 cup of beef stock every hour.

4. Slice the onion and place in a cast iron skillet, then pour the remaining cup of stock over the onions and set roast on top of onions.

5. Increase temperature to 275° F and cook an additional 2 ½ to 3 hours, or until internal temperature reaches 165° F.

6. Cover the roast with a cast iron lid or aluminum foil, and cook for another 2 ½ to 3

hours, or until the internal temperature reaches 200° F.

7. Remove chuck roast from the grill. Allow the roast to rest for 10 minutes, then remove from the skillet and shred.

8. Serve pulled roast beef in a hoagie roll with braised onions and pan jus.

Cheesy Skillet Shepherd's Pie

Servings: 4 - 6
Cooking Time: 40 Minutes

Ingredients:

- 2 Tbsp All-Purpose Flour
- 1 Cup Beef Broth
- ½ Tsp Black Pepper
- 2 Tbsp Butter
- 1 Cup Cheddar Cheese, Grated
- 4 Oz. Cream Cheese
- 3 Garlic Cloves, Minced
- 1 Lb. Ground Beef
- 1 Tbsp Italian Parsley
- 1 Tbsp Kosher Salt
- 1 Tbsp Olive Oil
- ½ Cup Minced Onion
- 1 ½ Cup Peas, Frozen
- 2 Tsp Pulled Pork Rub
- 1 Tsp Rosemary, Finely Chopped
- 1 ½ Lbs. Russet Potatoes, Peeled And Quartered

Directions:

1. Supply your smoker with wood pellets and follow the start-up procedure. Preheat the grill, with the lid closed, to 400° F. If using a gas or charcoal grill, set the temp to medium-high heat.

2. In a cast iron Dutch oven, bring potatoes and just enough water to cover to a boil. Add salt and cook until tender, 12 to 15 minutes. Drain potatoes, and return to pot. Add cream cheese, butter, ½ teaspoon salt, ½ teaspoon black pepper, and mash until smooth. Set aside.

3. Place cast iron skillet on grill and heat oil. Add onion and sauté 2 minutes, then add garlic and sauté until fragrant. Add ground beef, Pulled Pork Rub, and rosemary, and cook, stirring occasionally, breaking up the meat until browned.

4. Sprinkle flour over beef and stir until combined. Add the broth and cook, stirring until thickened, about 3 minutes.

5. Add a layer of peas over beef and sprinkle with parsley. Dollop mashed potatoes on top of peas and spread evenly.

6. Increase temperature to 450° F. Cover and cook for 5 minutes, then top with grated cheese. Cover and cook and additional 5 to 7 minutes, until cheese is melted, and edges of potatoes begin to brown. Serve hot.

Traeger Smoked Salami

Servings: 8
Cooking Time: 480 Minutes

Ingredients:

- Pound Ground Sirloin
- 1 Tablespoon Morton Tender Quick Home Meat Cure
- Tablespoon Worcestershire sauce
- 1 Tablespoon ground black pepper
- 2 Teaspoon mustard seeds
- 1 Teaspoon red pepper flakes
- 1 Teaspoon black peppercorn
- Teaspoon honey

Directions:

1. Plan ahead! This recipe requires overnight time. In a large glass bowl combine the beef, curing salt, Worcestershire, pepper, mustard, red

pepper flakes, and peppercorns. Gently distribute the ingredients through the meat.

2. Cover with plastic wrap and refrigerate for 1 day.

3. After the meat has cured for 1 day, lay two pieces of long plastic wrap on top of each other on your work surface. Overturn the meat directly into the middle of the plastic wrap. Form the meat into a long log shape.

4. Pull the plastic wrap around one side and smooth out the edges of the log. Use even pressure across the length to work out any bubbles. Pull the plastic wrap tightly around the other side and overlap the edges of the wrap to create a tight seal. Roll the sausage forward and back with both hands. Once you have the sausage fairly uniform in width, tightly twist the ends of the plastic wrap. Return to the refrigerator for 1 day.

5. Supply your smoker with wood pellets and follow the start-up procedure. Preheat the grill, with the lid closed, to 180° F.

6. Unwrap the sausage and drizzle with the honey. Place directly on the grill grate, close the lid and smoke for 6-8 hours or until the internal temperature of the sausage reads 170℉ with a meat thermometer. Probe: 170 ℉

7. Allow the sausage to cool completely before slicing and serving. Enjoy!

Bison Meatballs

Servings: 8 - 10

Cooking Time: 30 Minutes

Ingredients:

- ➢ 1 Cored, Peeled, And Chopped Apple
- ➢ 2 Tablespoons Beef & Brisket Rub
- ➢ 2 Cups Beef Broth
- ➢ 2 Pounds Ground Bison
- ➢ ¼ Cup Breadcrumbs
- ➢ 3 Tablespoons Cornstarch
- ➢ 2 Tablespoons Dijon Mustard
- ➢ 2 Beaten Eggs
- ➢ 1 Finely Garlic Clove, Minced
- ➢ 2 Cups Hard Cider
- ➢ 3 Tablespoons Pure Maple Syrup
- ➢ 2 Tablespoons Olive Oil
- ➢ ½ Cup Pureed Onion
- ➢ ¼ Pound Pancetta
- ➢ 3 Tablespoons Water
- ➢ 1 Thinly Sliced Yellow Onion

Directions:

1. First, make the mustard sauce. In a large saucepan, add the olive oil over medium heat, then add the onion and apple. Cook the apple and onion until soft and caramelized, about 10-12 minutes. Once the onion and apple are soft, add in the hard cider, beef broth, maple syrup and Dijon mustard to the pan. Whisk everything together and bring the sauce to a boil.

2. Once the sauce comes to a boil, reduce it to a simmer and cook, stirring and scraping the bottom of the pot occasionally until the sauce reduces by half, about 30 minutes. Remove the sauce from the heat and allow it to cool.

3. Pour the sauce into a blender, place the lid on top, and blend the sauce until completely smooth. Return the sauce into the saucepan and bring it back to a boil. In a small bowl, mix together the cornstarch and water, then pour into the sauce. Cook the sauce until thickened, whisking the entire time, about 2 minutes. Set the sauce aside.

4. Make the meatballs. In a food processor, blend the pancetta until it becomes a smooth paste. Scrape the pancetta into large mixing bowl,

and mix it with the ground bison, pureed onion, eggs, breadcrumbs, garlic, and Beef and Brisket Rub. Gently mix the meat together and, using a cookie scoop, scoop into meatballs. Place the meatballs on a baking sheet. Repeat with the remaining meat mixture.

5. Supply your smoker with wood pellets and follow the start-up procedure. Preheat the grill, with the lid closed, to 350° F. If you're using a gas or charcoal grill, set it up for medium heat. Place a large cast iron skillet on the grill and add the olive oil to it. Place the meatballs in an even layer in the skillet and grill, turning the meatballs occasionally until they are browned on all sides. Insert a temperature probe into one of the meatballs and continue grilling them until the internal temperature reaches 160°F.

6. Remove the meatballs from the grill, toss them with the mustard sauce, and serve immediately.

Savory Smoked Brisket

Servings: 10
Cooking Time: 600 Minutes

Ingredients:
- 4 Tbsp Apple Cider Vinegar
- 10Lb Trimmed Brisket
- 2 Cups Broth, Beef
- Sweet Heat Rub
- 2 Tbsp Worcestershire Sauce

Directions:
1. Trim the fat cap from your brisket, leaving enough fat to baste the meat during the smoke process.
2. Generously coat the brisket with Sweet Heat rub, and massage into the brisket.

3. In a bowl, whisk together the apple cider vinegar, Worcestershire sauce and beef broth, then pour into a clean spray bottle.

4. Supply your smoker with wood pellets and follow the start-up procedure. Preheat the grill, with the lid closed, to 225° F. Once the smoker is up to temperature, place the brisket inside and insert the temperature probe. Smoke for 10 to 12 hours, or until the internal temperature of the brisket reaches 200°F at the thickest part. Once an hour, spray the brisket with the mop sauce to baste it.

5. Once the brisket is done, remove from the smoker, allow to rest for 30 minutes under tin foil, then slice and enjoy!

Roasted Venison Steaks By The Bowmars

Servings: 4
Cooking Time: 25 Minutes

Ingredients:
- 10 Whole Venison Steaks, 6oz
- 1 L Diet Sprite
- 6 Ounce Big Game Rub
- 2 Pound asparagus
- 3 Tablespoon Rub

Directions:
1. The night before, marinade the steaks with sprite and big game rub.
2. Supply your smoker with wood pellets and follow the start-up procedure. Preheat the grill, with the lid closed, to 350° F.
3. Remove steaks from marinade and pat dry. Place steaks directly on the grill grate and cook 10-15 minutes flipping once until the internal temperature reaches 125 degrees for medium rare. Grill: 350 °F

4. Sprinkle asparagus with Traeger Rub and add to Traeger. Cook for 10 minutes turning once.

5. Let steaks rest ten minutes before serving. Enjoy!

Flavour Smoked Corned Beef Brisket Hash

Servings: 4

Cooking Time: 195 Minutes

Ingredients:

- 6 slices, chopped bacon
- 1 tsp black pepper
- 2 cups chicken stock
- 1, 2 lb. corned beef brisket
- 2 tbsp Italian parsley
- 1 ½ tsp hickory bacon rub
- 1, chopped red bell pepper
- 1 tsp thyme, fresh, chopped
- 1, chopped yellow onion
- 1 ½ lbs yukon gold potatoes

Directions:

1. Remove corned beef brisket from packaging, rinse under cold water, and pat dry with paper towel.

2. Season brisket with included seasoning packet and coarse black pepper, then rest for 30 minutes.

3. Supply your smoker with wood pellets and follow the start-up procedure. Preheat the grill, with the lid closed, to 225° F. If using a gas or charcoal grill, set it up for low indirect heat.

4. Lay brisket directly on the grill grate and smoke for 2 ½ to 3 hours or until the internal temperature reaches 165°F.

5. Once this temperature is achieved, place the brisket in a 9 x 13 metal pan with potatoes and chicken stock.

6. Cover with foil and cook until brisket reaches an internal temperature of 202°F.

7. Remove brisket from grill and refrigerate overnight or until brisket and potatoes have fully cooled.

8. When ready to cook, peel and dice potatoes then chop up 1 lb. of brisket, reserving the remainder for future use.

9. Place a cast-iron skillet on the pellet grill and preheat to 400°F.

10. Once skillet is heated, add bacon and sauté for 8 to 10 minutes, until brown.

11. Remove with slotted spoon and place on paper towel-lined tray.

12. Add onion and red bell pepper to skillet with rendered bacon fat and sauté for 3 minutes, then add cooked brisket.

13. Add Hickory Bacon Rub, parsley and thyme and sauté another 3 minutes.

14. Add diced potatoes. Gently stir to incorporate and serve hot.

Texas-style Smoked Beef Brisket By Doug Scheiding

Servings: 6

Cooking Time: 1080 Minutes

Ingredients:

- 1 (12-15 lb) brisket
- 2/3 Cup Butcher BBQ Prime Brisket Injection
- 2 Cup water
- 2 Tablespoon canola oil
- 1 1/2 Cup apple juice
- 1 Cup Prime Rib Rub
- 1 Cup Coffee Rub
- 4 Tablespoon ground black pepper

Directions:

1. Trim fat cap off the top of brisket and remove all silverskin. Trim off any brown areas such as on the side of the brisket. Make a long cut with the grain on the flat (thin side) of the brisket and a short cut again on the flat to show direction of cuts after cooking. Trim bottom fat cap to about 1/4 inch thickness.

2. Combine Butcher BBQ Prime Brisket Injection and water. Inject into the brisket with the grain in a checkerboard fashion. Rub entire brisket with canola oil then spritz with apple juice and let sit for 30 minutes.

3. Combine both Traeger rubs and season brisket liberally. Season the top with the black pepper.

4. Supply your smoker with wood pellets and follow the start-up procedure. Preheat the grill, with the lid closed, to 180° F.

5. Place brisket directly on the grill grate and cook 8 to 12 hours fat side down. Spritz with apple juice every 30 to 45 minutes after the first 3 hours. Grill: 180 ˚F Probe: 160 ˚F

6. After 8 hours, begin taking the temperature by inserting about two-thirds of the way up into the thickest part. It should register between 150˚F to 160˚F. Once the brisket registers 160˚F, wrap with two sheets of aluminum foil leaving one end open. Pour in remaining brisket injection and seal foil packet. Increase the temperature on the grill to 225˚F and place wrapped brisket directly on grill grate. Cook for another 3 to 4 hours until internal temperature registers 204˚F. Grill: 225 ˚F Probe: 204 ˚F

7. Remove from the grill and place in a cooler wrapped in a towel to rest for at least 2 hours. When ready to serve, cut slices about the thickness of a pencil against the grain. If desired, separate cooking liquid from fat and pour juices over cut slices of brisket. Enjoy!

Smoked Meatball Egg Sandwiches

Servings: 4

Cooking Time: 25 Minutes

Ingredients:
- 3/4 Cup Breadcrumbs
- 2 Cloves Garlic, Minced
- 1 & 1/2 Lb. Ground Chuck
- 1 Jar Of Your Favorite Marinara Sauce
- 1 Large Eggs
- ¼ Cup Onion
- ¼ Cup Parsley, Minced Fresh
- ½ Tsp Pepper
- 1 Tbsp Chop House Steak Seasoning
- Provolone Cheese, Sliced
- ½ Tsp Salt
- Shredded Mozzarella Cheese
- 4 Sub Rolls Or Baguettes (6"), Sliced
- 2 Tbsp Worcestershire

Directions:
1. In a larger mixing bowl, combine the ground chuck, onions, garlic, Chop House Steak seasoning, salt, pepper, fresh parsley, Worcestershire, and egg. Add the breadcrumb mixture and parmesan cheese to the bowl and fold it into meat until well combined.

2. Supply your smoker with wood pellets and follow the start-up procedure. Preheat the grill, with the lid closed, to 400° F. If you're using a gas or charcoal grill, set it up for medium high heat and add your cast iron pan to the grill to warm up.

3. Roll the meat mixture into balls about 1 ½ inches wide, roughly the size of golf balls. Place meatballs into the cast iron skillet. Cook for 15

minutes or until meatballs are fully cooked and beginning to brown.

4.   Pour full jar of marinara into the cast iron pan and gently stir to coat meatballs. Let simmer for 10-15 minutes.

5.   Tear off four sheets of aluminum foil and place a sliced bun in the center of each. Divide the meatballs with sauce among the rolls. Top each roll with provolone cheese slices and mozzarella, and wrap entire sandwich tightly in foil. Return to the grill and cook an additional 10 minutes or until cheese is melty and bread has toasted. Serve immediately and enjoy!

Citrus Grilled Lamb Chops

Servings: 4 - 6
Cooking Time: 15 Minutes

Ingredients:

➢ 2 Tablespoons Chophouse Steak Seasoning
➢ 4 Finely Garlic Clove, Minced
➢ 2 Pounds Thick Cut Rib Chops Or Lamb Loin
➢ Juice From 1/2 Lemon
➢ Juice From 1/2 Lime
➢ ¼ Cup Olive Oil
➢ 3 Tablespoons Orange Juice
➢ ¼ Cup Red Wine Vinegar

Directions:

1.   In a mixing bowl, whisk together all the ingredients and 2 tbsp Chophouse Steak. Place the lamb chops in a glass baking pan and pour the marinade over the top. Flip the chops over a few times to make sure that they are completely coated.

2.   Cover the glass pan in aluminum foil and allow the lamb chops to marinade for 4-12 hours.

Once the meat has finished marinating, drain off the excess marinade and discard.

3.   Supply your smoker with wood pellets and follow the start-up procedure. Preheat the grill, with the lid closed, to 400° F. If you're using a gas or charcoal grill, set it up for medium high heat. Grill the chops for 5-7 minutes per side, then lower the temperature to 350°F or medium heat, and flip and grill for another 5-7 minutes.

4.   Remove the lamb chops from the grill, cover in foil, and allow to rest for 5 minutes before serving.

Smoked Beef Back Ribs

Servings: 6
Cooking Time: 480 Minutes

Ingredients:

➢ 2 Rack beef back ribs
➢ 1/2 Cup Beef Rub

Directions:

1.   If your butcher has not already done so, remove the thin papery membrane from the bone-side of the ribs by working the tip of a butter knife underneath the membrane over a middle bone. Use paper towels to get a firm grip, then tear the membrane off.

2.   Season both sides of ribs with Traeger Beef Rub.

3.   Supply your smoker with wood pellets and follow the start-up procedure. Preheat the grill, with the lid closed, to 225° F.

4.   Arrange the ribs on the grill grate, bone side down. Cook for 8-10 hours, or until internal temperature reaches 205°F. Grill: 225 °F Probe: 205 °F

5. Remove ribs from grill and let rest, lightly covered for 20 minutes before slicing and serving. Enjoy!

Traeger Bbq Brisket

Servings: 8
Cooking Time: 540 Minutes

Ingredients:
- 1 (12-14 lb) whole packer brisket, trimmed
- Beef Rub

Directions:
1. Coat meat liberally with Traeger Beef Rub. When seasoned, wrap brisket in plastic wrap. Transfer wrapped brisket to the refrigerator and let sit for 12 to 24 hours.
2. Supply your smoker with wood pellets and follow the start-up procedure. Preheat the grill, with the lid closed, to 225° F.
3. Remove brisket from plastic wrap and place fat side down on the grill grate. Cook for 6 hours or until internal temperature reaches 160°F. Grill: 225 °F Probe: 160 °F
4. Remove brisket from the grill and wrap in a double layer of foil.
5. Place foiled brisket back on grill and cook until it reaches a finished internal temperature of 204°F, this should take an additional 3 to 4 hours. Grill: 225 °F Probe: 204 °F
6. Remove from grill and rest in the foil for at least 30 minutes. Slice against the grain. Enjoy!

Spatchcocked Quail With Smoked Fruit

Servings: 4
Cooking Time: 60 Minutes

Ingredients:
- 4 quail, spatchcocked
- 2 teaspoons salt
- 2 teaspoons freshly ground black pepper
- 2 teaspoons garlic powder
- 4 ripe peaches or pears
- 4 tablespoons (½ stick) salted butter, softened
- 1 tablespoon sugar
- 1 teaspoon ground cinnamon

Directions:
1. Supply your smoker with wood pellets and follow the start-up procedure. Preheat, with the lid closed, to 225°F.
2. Season the quail all over with the salt, pepper, and garlic powder.
3. Cut the peaches (or pears) in half and remove the pits (or the cores).
4. In a small bowl, combine the butter, sugar, and cinnamon; set aside.
5. Arrange the quail on the grill grate, close the lid, and smoke for about 1 hour, or until a meat thermometer inserted in the thickest part reads 145°F.
6. After the quail has been cooking for about 15 minutes, add the peaches (or pears) to the grill, flesh-side down, and smoke for 30 to 40 minutes.
7. Top the cooked peaches (or pears) with the cinnamon butter and serve alongside the quail.

Cheese Onion Steak Sandwiches

Servings: 4
Cooking Time: 10 Minutes

Ingredients:
- 2 tbsp, divided butter
- 4 hoagie rolls, sliced lengthwise
- 2 tbsp olive oil
- 1-2 tbsp chop house steak rub
- 8 slices provolone cheese, sliced

- ➢ 2 lbs, sliced thinly rib-eye steaks
- ➢ 1 yellow onion, sliced

Directions:

1. Supply your smoker with wood pellets and follow the start-up procedure. Preheat the grill, with the lid closed, to 375° F. If using a gas or charcoal grill, set heat to medium heat. For all other grills, preheat cast iron skillet on grill grates.

2. Melt 1 tablespoon of butter and 1 tablespoon of olive oil on griddle. With a serrated knife, slice rolls 3/4 of the way through, then place facedown onto griddle and cook until toasted. Set aside.

3. Melt remaining tablespoon of butter and olive oil on the griddle. Add sliced onions and cook for 2 minutes, or until lightly caramelized. Move to the lower-right corner of griddle to keep warm.

4. Season steak generously with Chop House Steak Rub, then place on griddle and cook for 3 minutes, stirring to brown all sides. Mix in caramelized onions.

5. Divide steak and onions into 4 portions on the griddle, then top each with 2 slices of provolone cheese. Let cheese melt slightly and transfer to a toasted hoagie roll using a bench scraper or metal spatula. Serve hot and enjoy!

Chorizo Cheese Stuffed Burgers

Servings: 2

Cooking Time: 45 Minutes

Ingredients:

- ➢ 2 Pound ground beef, 80% lean
- ➢ 4 Ounce Prime Rib Rub
- ➢ 12 Ounce Chorizo
- ➢ 2 Slices cheddar cheese
- ➢ 4 Whole Brioche Bun
- ➢ Tomatoes, sliced
- ➢ red onion, sliced

- ➢ lettuce, sliced

Directions:

1. Mix 2 lb of 80/20 ground beef in mixing bowl with Traeger Prime Rib Rub.

2. Divide the ground beef into eight 1/4 lb patties. Make one patty the base, lay down 1/4 of a cheese slice, add 3 oz. of chorizo and top with another 1/4 cheese slice. Apply another patty on top and pinch the ends all the way around the burger to seal together the two patties.

3. Repeat until all 4 patties are done.

4. Supply your smoker with wood pellets and follow the start-up procedure. Preheat the grill, with the lid closed, to 325° F.

5. Place burgers on the Traeger for 15 minutes on each side. If desired, top each burger with slice of Cheddar cheese, let melt. Remove from Traeger and let rest for 10 minutes tented with foil.

6. While burgers are resting, brush the brioche buns with melted better and toast for 30-45 seconds on the grill.

7. Remove buns from grill and assemble burger with toppings. Enjoy!

Spicy Smoked Chili Beef Jerky

Servings: 6

Cooking Time: 240 Minutes

Ingredients:

- ➢ 1 Cup chili sauce
- ➢ 1/3 Cup beer
- ➢ 2 Tablespoon soy sauce
- ➢ 1 Tablespoon Worcestershire sauce
- ➢ 2 Tablespoon Morton Tender Quick Home Meat Cure
- ➢ 1 Tablespoon minced pickled jalapeño peppers

➢ 2 Pound flank steak, cut into 1/4 inch thick slices

Directions:

1. In a mixing bowl, combine the chili sauce, beer, soy sauce, Worcestershire sauce, curing salt and pickled jalapeño peppers.

2. Put the beef slices in a large resealable bag. Pour the marinade mixture over the beef, and massage the bag so that all the slices get coated with the marinade. Seal the bag and refrigerate for several hours, or overnight.

3. Supply your smoker with wood pellets and follow the start-up procedure. Preheat the grill, with the lid closed, to 165° F.

4. Remove the beef from the marinade, discarding the marinade. Dry beef slices between paper towels.

5. Arrange the meat in a single layer directly on the grill grate or smoke shelf.

6. Smoke for 4 to 5 hours, or until the jerky is dry but still chewy and somewhat pliant when bending a piece. Grill: 165 °F

7. Transfer to a resealable bag while the jerky is still warm.

8. Let the jerky rest for an hour at room temperature. Squeeze any air from the bag, and refrigerate the jerky.

9. Pro Tip: you can use this recipe for any cut of beef or wild game. Enjoy!

Baked Maple Venison Sausage Quiche

Servings: 4
Cooking Time: 45 Minutes

Ingredients:
➢ 2 Pound Venison, ground
➢ 12 Whole egg
➢ 16 Ounce Cottage Cheese, fat free
➢ 1 1/2 Cup Cheese, Colby/Cheddar
➢ 1 Teaspoon baking powder
➢ 1 Whole white onion, chopped
➢ 4 Ounce Green Chiles, canned, chopped

Directions:

1. Cook ground venison in a medium sauté pan over medium high until browned. Drain off excess fat and set venison aside.

2. Whisk eggs in a large mixing bowl. Add remaining ingredients, stirring after each addition. Transfer mixture to one 13x9 pan and one 9x9 pan.

3. Supply your smoker with wood pellets and follow the start-up procedure. Preheat the grill, with the lid closed, to 350° F.

4. Place casserole dish directly on grill grate and cook for 45 minutes or until a knife inserted into the center comes out clean. Let cool 10 minutes before serving. Enjoy!

5. This recipe was provided by Pro Team member Josh and Sarah Bowmar. Access this, and over a thousand other Traeger recipes on the Traeger App.

Greek Leg Of Lamb

Servings: 12-16
Cooking Time: 25 Minutes

Ingredients:
➢ 2 tablespoons finely chopped fresh rosemary
➢ 1 tablespoon ground thyme
➢ 5 garlic cloves, minced
➢ 2 tablespoons sea salt
➢ 1 tablespoon freshly ground black pepper
➢ Butcher's string
➢ 1 whole boneless (6- to 8-pound) leg of lamb
➢ ¼ cup extra-virgin olive oil

➢ 1 cup red wine vinegar

➢ ½ cup canola oil

Directions:

1. In a small bowl, combine the rosemary, thyme, garlic, salt, and pepper; set aside.

2. Using butcher's string, tie the leg of lamb into the shape of a roast. Your butcher should also be happy to truss the leg for you.

3. Rub the lamb generously with the olive oil and season with the spice mixture. Transfer to a plate, cover with plastic wrap, and refrigerate for 4 hours.

4. Remove the lamb from the refrigerator but do not rinse.

5. Supply your smoker with wood pellets and follow the start-up procedure. Preheat, with the lid closed, to 325°F.

6. In a small bowl, combine the red wine vinegar and canola oil for basting.

7. Place the lamb directly on the grill, close the lid, and smoke for 20 to 25 minutes per pound (depending on desired doneness), basting with the oil and vinegar mixture every 30 minutes. Lamb is generally served medium-rare to medium, so it will be done when a meat thermometer inserted in the thickest part reads 140°F to 145°F.

8. Let the lamb rest for about 15 minutes before slicing to serve.

COCKTAILS RECIPES

Smoked Salted Caramel White Russian

Servings: 4
Cooking Time: 20 Minutes

Ingredients:

- 16 Ounce half-and-half
- salted caramel sauce
- 6 Ounce vodka
- 6 Ounce Kahlúa

Directions:

1. Supply your smoker with wood pellets and follow the start-up procedure. Preheat the grill, with the lid closed, to 180° F.
2. Pour the half-and-half in a shallow baking dish and place directly on the grill grate. In another shallow baking dish, pour 2 to 3 cups of water and place on the grill next to the half-and-half.
3. Smoke both the half-and-half and water for 20 minutes. Remove from the grill and let cool. Grill: 180 ℉
4. Place the half-and-half in the fridge until ready to use. Pour the smoked water into ice cube trays and transfer to the freezer until completely frozen.
5. Separate the smoked ice cubes into four glasses. Drizzle the salted caramel sauce around the inside of the glass.
6. Pour 1-1/2 ounce vodka and 1-1/2 ounce Kahlúa into each of the glasses and top with the smoked half-and-half. Enjoy!

Traeger Boulevardier Cocktail

Servings: 2
Cooking Time: 60 Minutes

Ingredients:

- 4 oranges
- 1/2 Cup honey
- 1500 mL rye whiskey
- 1 1/2 Ounce Campari
- 1 1/2 Ounce sweet vermouth
- 2 Tablespoon granulated sugar
- 3 Ounce grilled orange infused rye

Directions:

1. Supply your smoker with wood pellets and follow the start-up procedure. Preheat the grill, with the lid closed, to 350° F.
2. Slice 2 oranges in half and coat cut side with honey. Peel remaining orange and place peels on the grill. Cook 20 to 25 minutes. Grill: 350 ℉
3. Remove from grill and let cool. Place orange halves cut side down directly on the grill grate and cook 20 to 30 minutes or until dark grill marks appear. Remove orange halves and allow to cool. Grill: 350 ℉
4. Place orange halves into a bottle of rye whiskey and let steep for 10 to 12 hours. The longer they steep, the sweeter and more pronounced the orange flavor will be.
5. Add all ingredients into a mixing glass and stir until diluted. Strain into a fresh coupe glass and serve neat.
6. Garnish with grilled orange peel. Enjoy!

Garden Gimlet Cocktail

Servings: 2
Cooking Time: 45 Minutes

Ingredients:

- 2 Cup honey
- 4 lemons, zested
- 4 Sprig rosemary, plus more for garnish
- 1/2 Cup water
- 4 Slices cucumber
- 1 1/2 Ounce lime juice
- 3 Ounce vodka

Directions:

1. Supply your smoker with wood pellets and follow the start-up procedure. Preheat the grill, with the lid closed, to 180° F.
2. To make smoked lemon and rosemary honey syrup, thin 1 cup honey by adding 1/4 cup water to a shallow pan. Add lemon zest and 2 sprigs rosemary.
3. Place the pan directly on the grill grate and smoke 45 minutes to an hour. Remove from heat, strain and cool. Grill: 180 ˚F
4. In a cocktail shaker, muddle the cucumbers and 1oz of the smoked lemon and rosemary honey syrup.
5. After muddling, add lime juice, vodka, and ice. Shake and double strain into a coup glass.
6. Garnish with a sprig of rosemary. Enjoy!

Zombie Cocktail Recipe

Servings: 2
Cooking Time: 45 Minutes

Ingredients:

- fresh squeezed orange juice
- pineapple juice
- 2 Ounce light rum
- 2 Ounce dark rum
- 2 Ounce lime juice
- 1 Ounce Smoked Simple Syrup
- 6 Ounce smoked orange and pineapple juice
- 2 grilled orange peel, for garnish
- 2 grilled pineapple chunks, for garnish

Directions:

1. Supply your smoker with wood pellets and follow the start-up procedure. Preheat the grill, with the lid closed, to 180° F.
2. Smoked Orange and Pineapple Juice: Pour equal parts fresh squeezed orange juice and pineapple juice into a shallow sheet pan and smoke for 45 minutes. Remove and let cool. Measure out 3 ounces of juice and reserve any remaining juice in the refrigerator for future use. Grill: 180 ˚F
3. Add dark and light rums, 3 ounces smoked orange and pineapple juice, lime juice and Traeger Smoked Simple Syrup to a mixing glass.
4. Add ice, shake and strain over clean ice into a Tiki glass.
5. Garnish with a grilled orange peel and grilled pineapple. Enjoy!

Traeger Smoked Daiquiri

Servings: 2
Cooking Time: 25 Minutes

Ingredients:

- 2 limes, sliced
- 2 Tablespoon granulated sugar
- 3 Ounce Rum
- 1 Ounce Smoked Simple Syrup
- 1 1/2 Ounce lime juice

Directions:

1. Supply your smoker with wood pellets and follow the start-up procedure. Preheat the grill, with the lid closed, to 350° F.

2. Toss the lime slices with granulated sugar and place directly on the grill grate. Cook 20-25 minutes or until grill marks form. Remove from grill and cool. Grill: 350 ˚F

3. In a mixing glass add rum, Traeger Simple Syrup, and fresh lime juice. Add ice to the mixing glass and shake. Strain contents into a chilled glass.

4. Garnish with a grilled lime wheel. Enjoy!

Smoked Irish Coffee

Servings: 2

Cooking Time: 15 Minutes

Ingredients:

➢ 10 Ounce hot coffee

➢ 1/2 Cup heavy cream

➢ 1 Tablespoon sugar

➢ 2 Ounce Irish whiskey

➢ freshly grated nutmeg, for garnish (optional)

Directions:

1. Supply your smoker with wood pellets and follow the start-up procedure. Preheat the grill, with the lid closed, to 180° F.

2. Place the coffee and cream in separate shallow baking dishes and place both directly on the grill grate. Smoke for 10 to 15 minutes until the liquids pick up a slight smoke flavor. Grill: 180 ˚F

3. Remove from the grill and cool the cream. When the cream is cool, add sugar and whip in a stand mixer or by hand to soft peaks.

4. Pour the hot coffee into two mugs then add 2 ounces of whiskey to each.

5. Top with smoked whipped cream and finish with freshly grated nutmeg, if desired. Enjoy!

Smoked Plum And Thyme Fizz Cocktail

Servings: 2

Cooking Time: 60 Minutes

Ingredients:

➢ 6 fresh plums

➢ 4 Fluid Ounce vodka

➢ 1 1/2 Fluid Ounce fresh lemon juice

➢ 2 Ounce smoked plum and thyme simple syrup

➢ 4 Fluid Ounce club soda

➢ 2 Slices smoked plum, for garnish

➢ 2 Sprig fresh thyme, for garnish

➢ 8 Sprig thyme

➢ 2 Cup Smoked Simple Syrup

Directions:

1. Supply your smoker with wood pellets and follow the start-up procedure. Preheat the grill, with the lid closed, to 180° F.

2. Cut plums in half and remove the pit. Place the plum halves directly on the grill grate and smoke for 25 minutes. Grill: 180 ˚F

3. For the Plum and Thyme Simple Syrup: After 25 minutes, remove plums from the grill and cut into quarters. Add plums and thyme sprigs to 1 cup of Traeger Smoked Simple Syrup. Smoke the mixture for 45 minutes. Remove from grill, strain and let cool. Grill: 180 ˚F

4. Add vodka, fresh lemon juice and smoked plum and thyme simple syrup to a mixing glass.

5. Add ice and shake. Strain over clean ice, top off with club soda and garnish with a piece of thyme and slice of smoked plum. Enjoy!

Sunset Margarita

Servings: 2
Cooking Time: 55 Minutes

Ingredients:

➢ 4 oranges
➢ 2 Cup plus 1 teaspoon agave
➢ 1/2 Cup water
➢ 1 Ounce burnt orange agave
➢ 3 Ounce reposado tequila
➢ 1 1/2 Ounce fresh squeezed lime juice
➢ Jacobsen Salt Co. Cherrywood Smoked Salt

Directions:

1. Supply your smoker with wood pellets and follow the start-up procedure. Preheat the grill, with the lid closed, to 350° F.

2. For the Burnt Orange Agave Syrup: Cut one orange in half and brush cut side with agave. Place cut side down directly on the grill grate and grill for 15 minutes or until grill marks develop. Grill: 350 °F

3. While the orange halves are grilling, slice the other orange and brush both sides of the slices with agave. Place slices directly on the grill grate next to the halves and cook for 15 minutes or until grill marks develop. Grill: 350 °F

4. Remove orange halves from grill grate and let cool. After they have cooled, juice halves and strain. Set aside.

5. Combine 1/4 cup water and agave in a shallow dish and mix well. Remove orange slices from the grill and place in the agave mixture, reserving a few for garnish.

6. Reduce the grill temperature to 180 degrees F and place the shallow dish with agave and oranges directly on the grill grate. Smoke for 40 minutes. Remove from heat and strain. Set aside. Grill: 180 °F

7. To Mix Drink: Rim glass with Jacobsen Smoked Salt. Combine tequila, fresh lime juice, grilled orange juice and burnt orange agave syrup in a glass. Add ice and shake well.

8. Strain into a rimmed glass over clean ice. Garnish with a grilled orange slice. Enjoy!

Smoked Pomegranate Lemonade Cocktail

Servings: 2
Cooking Time: 45 Minutes

Ingredients:

➢ 32 Ounce POM Juice
➢ 2 Cup pomegranate seeds
➢ 3 Ounce vodka
➢ 8 Ounce lemonade
➢ lemon wheel, for garnish
➢ fresh mint, for garnish

Directions:

1. Supply your smoker with wood pellets and follow the start-up procedure. Preheat the grill, with the lid closed, to 225° F.

2. For the Smoked Pomegranate Ice Cubes: Pour one small container of POM juice and 1 cup of pomegranate seeds into a shallow sheet pan. Smoke on the Traeger for 45 minutes. Pull off grill and let sit until cooled. Grill: 180 °F

3. Pour smoked POM juice into ice molds of your choice and put into freezer.

4. When ready to serve, place the frozen pomegranate cubes into a mason jar. Pour vodka and lemonade over the ice cubes.

5. Garnish with a lemon wheel and fresh mint. Enjoy!

Smoked Hibiscus Sparkler

Servings: 4

Cooking Time: 30 Minutes

Ingredients:

- 1/2 Cup sugar
- 2 Tablespoon dried hibiscus flowers
- 1 Bottle sparkling wine
- crystallized ginger, for garnish

Directions:

1. Supply your smoker with wood pellets and follow the start-up procedure. Preheat the grill, with the lid closed, to 180° F.

2. Place water in a shallow baking dish and place directly on the grill grate. Smoke the water for 30 minutes or until desired smoke flavor is achieved. Grill: 180 °F

3. Pour water into a small saucepan and add sugar and hibiscus flowers. Bring to a simmer over medium heat and cook until sugar is dissolved.

4. Strain out the hibiscus flowers and transfer your simple syrup to a small container and refrigerate until chilled.

5. Pour 1/2 ounce smoked hibiscus simple syrup in the bottom of a champagne glass and top with sparkling wine.

6. Drop in a few pieces of crystallized ginger to garnish. Enjoy!

Smoked Pineapple Hotel Nacional Cocktail

Servings: 2

Cooking Time: 20 Minutes

Ingredients:

- 2 pineapple
- 1/2 Cup water
- 1/2 Cup sugar
- 3 Fluid Ounce white rum
- 1 1/2 Fluid Ounce lime juice
- 1 1/2 Fluid Ounce Pineapple Syrup
- 1 Fluid Ounce apricot brandy
- 2 Dash Angostura bitters

Directions:

1. For the Syrup: Supply your smoker with wood pellets and follow the start-up procedure. Preheat the grill, with the lid closed, to 180° F.

2. Trim both ends of the pineapple, discard the ends. Cut the pineapple into slices about 3/4" thick. Don't worry about the skin, it doesn't hurt to leave it on. Place the pineapple slices on the grill and smoke for about 15 minutes on each sideTrim both ends of the pineapple and discard the ends. Cut the pineapple into slices about 3/4 inch thick. Don't worry about the skin, it doesn't hurt to leave it on. Place the pineapple slices on the grill and smoke for about 15 minutes per side. Grill: 180 °F

3. While the pineapple is smoking, combine 1/4 cup water and sugar in a saucepan over low heat, stirring constantly, until sugar is dissolved. Pour syrup into a large bowl and set aside.

4. When the pineapple is done cooking, cut each slice into eight or so wedges and add the wedges to the bowl with the simple syrup, tossing to coat and cover.

5. Leave the mixture to macerate for at least 4 hours (or up to 24) in the refrigerator, stirring from time to time.

6. Strain the syrup into a clean bowl through a fine-mesh strainer and press on the pineapple with a ladle to extract as much liquid as possible. You can bottle and refrigerate the syrup for up to 4 days.

7. To make the cocktail: Combine the rum, lime juice, pineapple syrup, apricot brandy, and bitters in a cocktail shaker or mixing glass. Fill with ice cubes and shake until cold.

8. Strain into a chilled cocktail glass. Garnish with a lime wheel and serve. Enjoy!

Grilled Blood Orange Mimosa

Servings: 4
Cooking Time: 15 Minutes

Ingredients:
- 3 blood orange, halved
- 2 Tablespoon granulated sugar
- 1 Bottle sparkling wine
- thyme sprigs, for garnish

Directions:
1. Supply your smoker with wood pellets and follow the start-up procedure. Preheat the grill, with the lid closed, to 375° F.
2. When the grill is hot, dip the cut side of the orange halves in sugar and place cut side down directly on the grill grate. Grill: 375 ℉
3. Grill the oranges for 10-15 minutes or until grill marks develop. Grill: 375 ℉
4. Remove from the grill and let cool at room temperature.
5. When cool enough to handle, juice the oranges and strain through a fine strainer removing any pulp.
6. Pour 5 oz of sparkling wine into each glass and top with 1 oz blood orange juice.
7. Garnish with a sprig of thyme. Enjoy!

Strawberry Mule Cocktail

Servings: 2
Cooking Time: 15 Minutes

Ingredients:
- 8 grilled strawberries, plus more for serving
- 3 Ounce vodka
- 1 Ounce Smoked Simple Syrup
- 1 Ounce lemon juice
- 6 Ounce ginger beer
- fresh mint leaves

Directions:
1. Supply your smoker with wood pellets and follow the start-up procedure. Preheat the grill, with the lid closed, to 400° F.
2. Place strawberries directly on the grill grate and cook 15 minutes or until grill marks appear. Grill: 400 ℉
3. For the cocktail: Add vodka, grilled strawberries, Traeger Smoked Simple Syrup and lemon juice to a shaker. Shake vigorously.
4. Double strain into a fresh glass or copper mug with crushed ice.
5. Top with ginger beer and garnish with extra grilled strawberries and fresh mint. Enjoy!

Smoked Berry Cocktail

Servings: 2
Cooking Time: 15 Minutes

Ingredients:
- 1/2 Cup strawberries, stemmed
- 1/2 Cup blackberries
- 1/2 Cup blueberries
- 8 Ounce bourbon or iced tea
- 2 Ounce lime juice
- 3 Ounce simple syrup
- soda water
- fresh mint, for garnish

Directions:
1. Supply your smoker with wood pellets and follow the start-up procedure. Preheat the grill, with the lid closed, to 180° F.

2. Wash berries well, spread them on a clean cookie sheet and place on the grill. Smoke berries for 15 minutes. Grill: 180 ℉

3. Remove berries from grill and transfer to a blender. Puree berries until smooth then pass through a fine mesh strainer to remove seeds.

4. To create a layered cocktail, pour 2 ounces of berry puree in the bottom of a glass. Next, pour 2 ounces of bourbon or iced tea over the back of a spoon into the glass, then 1/2 ounce lime juice and 1/2 ounce simple syrup, top with soda water and ice. Finish with mint or extra berries for garnish.

5. Repeat the same process for 3 more servings. Enjoy!

Bacon Old-fashioned Cocktail

Servings: 2
Cooking Time: 20 Minutes

Ingredients:

- 16 Slices bacon
- 1/2 Cup warm water (110°F to 115°F)
- 1500 mL bourbon
- 1/2 Fluid Ounce maple syrup
- 4 Dash Angostura bitters
- 2 fresh orange peel

Directions:

1. Smoke bacon prior to making Old Fashioned using this recipe for Applewood Smoked Bacon.

2. To Make Bacon: Supply your smoker with wood pellets and follow the start-up procedure. Preheat the grill, with the lid closed, to 325° F.

3. Place bacon in a single layer on a cooling rack that fits inside a baking sheet pan. Cook in Traeger for 15-20 minutes or until bacon is browned and crispy. Reserve bacon for later. Let the fat cool slightly; you'll use the fat to infuse the bourbon. Grill: 325 ℉

4. Combine 1/4 cup of warm (not hot) liquid bacon fat with the entire contents of a 750ml bottle of bourbon in a glass or heavy plastic container.

5. Use a fork to stir well. Let it sit on the counter for a few hours, stirring every so often.

6. After about four hours, put bourbon fat mixture into the freezer. After about an hour, the fat will congeal and you can simply scoop it out with a spoon. You can fine-strain the mixture through a sieve to remove all fat if desired.

7. Combine ingredients with ice and stir until cold. Strain over fresh ice in an Old Fashioned glass and garnish with reserved bacon and orange peel. Enjoy!

Smoked Sangria

Servings: 6
Cooking Time: 45 Minutes

Ingredients:

- 1 (750 ml) medium-bodied red wine
- 1/4 Cup Grand Marnier
- 1/4 Cup Smoked Simple Syrup
- 1 Cup fresh cranberries
- 1 Whole apple, sliced
- 2 Whole limes, sliced
- 4 cinnamon stick
- soda water

Directions:

1. Supply your smoker with wood pellets and follow the start-up procedure. Preheat the grill, with the lid closed, to 180° F.

2. In a shallow dish, combine red wine, Grand Marnier, Traeger Smoked Simple Syrup and cranberries, and place directly on the grill grate.

3. Smoke for 30 to 45 minutes or until the liquid picks up desired amount of smoke. Remove from grill and place in the fridge to cool. Grill: 180 ℉

4. When the mixture has cooled, place in a large pitcher. Add sliced apples, limes, cinnamon sticks and ice to pitcher.

5. Top with soda water, if desired. Enjoy!

A Smoking Classic Cocktail

Servings: 2

Cooking Time: 60 Minutes

Ingredients:

- 2 Bottle Angostura orange bitters
- 10 sugar cubes
- 8 Ounce Champagne
- lemon twist

Directions:

1. Supply your smoker with wood pellets and follow the start-up procedure. Preheat the grill, with the lid closed, to 180° F.

2. For the Smoked Orange Bitters: In a small skillet, combine 1 bottle of Angostura orange bitters with a splash of water and 4 sugar cubes.

3. Place skillet on the grill grate and smoke for 60 minutes. Cool the smoked bitters and put back into the bottle. Grill: 180 ℉

4. Add a sugar cube to each Champagne flute and soak the sugar cubes with the smoked bitters.

5. Add champagne and a lemon twist in a flute glass. Enjoy!

Smoked Pumpkin Spice Latte

Servings: 4

Cooking Time: 45 Minutes

Ingredients:

- 1 Small sugar pumpkin
- olive oil
- 1 Can sweetened condensed milk
- 1 Cup whole milk
- 2 Tablespoon Smoked Simple Syrup
- 1 Teaspoon pumpkin pie spice
- pinch of salt
- cinnamon
- whipped cream
- shaved nutmeg
- 8 Ounce smoked cold brew coffee

Directions:

1. Supply your smoker with wood pellets and follow the start-up procedure. Preheat the grill, with the lid closed, to 325° F.

2. Cut the sugar pumpkin in half, scoop out the seeds and discard. Place the pumpkin halves cut side up on a baking sheet and brush lightly with olive oil.

3. Place the sheet tray directly on the grill grate and cook 45 minutes or until the flesh is tender. Remove from heat and place on the counter to cool. Grill: 325 ℉

4. When the pumpkin is cool enough to handle, scoop out the flesh and mash until smooth.

5. Place 3 Tbsp of the pumpkin puree in a separate bowl and reserve the remaining for another use.

6. Add the sweetened condensed milk, whole milk, Traeger Smoked Simple Syrup, pumpkin pie seasoning and salt to the pumpkin puree. Whisk to combine.

7. Pour the cold brew over ice, add desired amount of pumpkin spice creamer and top with whipped cream, cinnamon, and shaved nutmeg if desired. Enjoy!

Grilled Peach Smash Cocktail

Servings: 2

Cooking Time: 10 Minutes

Ingredients:

- ➤ 2 peach, sliced and grilled
- ➤ 10 fresh mint leaves
- ➤ 1 1/2 Ounce Smoked Simple Syrup
- ➤ 4 Ounce bourbon
- ➤ 2 mint sprig, for garnish

Directions:

1. Supply your smoker with wood pellets and follow the start-up procedure. Preheat the grill, with the lid closed, to 375° F.

2. Cut the peach into 6 slices and brush with Traeger Smoked Simple Syrup. Place directly on the grill grate and cook 10 to 12 minutes or until peaches soften and get grill marks. Grill: 375 ˚F

3. In a mixing glass, add 3 slices of grilled peaches, 5 mint leaves and Traeger Smoked Simple Syrup.

4. Muddle ingredients to release oils of the mint and juices from the grilled peaches. Add bourbon and crushed ice.

5. Shake and pour into a stemless wine glass. Top off with more crushed ice. Garnish with a grilled peach and mint sprig. Enjoy!

Smoke And Bubz Cocktail

Servings: 2

Cooking Time: 45 Minutes

Ingredients:

- ➤ 16 Ounce POM Juice
- ➤ 2 Cup pomegranate seeds
- ➤ 6 Ounce sparkling white wine
- ➤ 2 lemon twist, for garnish
- ➤ 2 Teaspoon pomegranate seeds

Directions:

1. Supply your smoker with wood pellets and follow the start-up procedure. Preheat the grill, with the lid closed, to 180° F.

2. For the Smoked Pomegranate Juice: Pour POM juice and a cup of pomegranate seeds into a shallow sheet pan. Smoke on the Traeger for 45 minutes. Pull off grill, strain, discard seeds and let sit until chilled. Grill: 180 ˚F

3. Add 1-1/2 ounces of the smoked pomegranate juice to the bottom of a champagne flute.

4. Add sparkling white wine, a few fresh pomegranate seeds and a lemon twist to garnish. Enjoy!

Batter Up Cocktail

Servings: 2

Cooking Time: 60 Minutes

Ingredients:

- ➤ 2 whole nutmeg
- ➤ 4 Ounce Michter's Bourbon
- ➤ 3 Teaspoon pumpkin puree
- ➤ 1 Ounce Smoked Simple Syrup
- ➤ 2 Large egg

Directions:

1. Supply your smoker with wood pellets and follow the start-up procedure. Preheat the grill, with the lid closed, to 180° F.

2. Place whole nutmeg on a sheet tray and place in the grill. Smoke 1 hour. Remove from grill and let cool. Grill: 180 ˚F

3. Add everything to a shaker and shake without ice. Add ice, then shake and strain into a chilled highball glass.

4. Garnish with grated, smoked nutmeg. Enjoy!

Grilled Frozen Strawberry Lemonade

Servings: 4

Cooking Time: 15 Minutes

Ingredients:

- 1 Pound fresh strawberries
- 1/2 Cup turbinado sugar
- 8 lemon, halved
- 1/4 Cup Cointreau
- 1/4 Cup simple syrup
- 2 Cup ice
- 1 Cup Titos Vodka

Directions:

1. Supply your smoker with wood pellets and follow the start-up procedure. Preheat the grill, with the lid closed, to High heat.

2. Dip the lemon halves in turbinado sugar and place directly on the grill grate. Toss the strawberries with remaining sugar and place next to the lemons.

3. Cook until grill marks develop on both, about 15 min for lemons and 10 min for strawberries.

4. Remove from heat and let cool.

5. Juice grilled lemons straining out any seeds or pulp. Pour into a blender pitcher.

6. Remove stems from grilled strawberries and place in blender pitcher with lemon juice. Add simple syrup, vodka, cointreau, and 2 cups of ice.

7. Puree until smooth and transfer to 4-6 glasses. Garnish with grilled strawberries and grilled lemon slices if desired. Enjoy!

Traeger Old Fashioned

Servings: 2

Cooking Time: 60 Minutes

Ingredients:

- 2 orange
- 2 Cup cherries
- 3 Ounce bourbon
- 1 Ounce Smoked Simple Syrup
- 8 Dash Bitters Lab Apricot Vanilla Bitters

Directions:

1. Supply your smoker with wood pellets and follow the start-up procedure. Preheat the grill, with the lid closed, to 180° F.

2. While Traeger preheats, slice whole orange into wheels.

3. Place cherries on a small sheet pan and place in the Traeger. Place orange slices directly on the grill grate.

4. Smoke cherries for 1 hour and oranges for 25 minutes, depending on taste, before removing from the grill. Let oranges and cherries cool. Grill: 180 °F

5. Pour bourbon into glass, followed by Traeger Smoked Simple Syrup and bitters. Add ice and stir for 45 seconds or until drink is well-diluted.

6. Strain contents into new glass over fresh ice. Skewer orange wheel and add cherry for garnish. Enjoy!

Printed by Libri Plureos GmbH in Hamburg, Germany